Neuropsychology of the Dreaming Brain

Neuropsychology of the Dreaming Brain

Kenneth D. Howell

iUniverse, Inc.

New York Lincoln Shanghai

Neuropsychology of the Dreaming Brain

iUniverse books may be ordered through booksellers or by contacting:

iUniverse
2021 Pine Lake Road, Suite 100
Lincoln, NE 68512
www.iuniverse.com
1-800-Authors (1-800-288-4677)

ISBN-13: 978-0-595-37261-4 (pbk)
ISBN-13: 978-0-595-81657-6 (ebk)
ISBN-10: 0-595-37261-9 (pbk)
ISBN-10: 0-595-81657-6 (ebk)

Printed in the United States of America

CONTENT

In the pages that follow I shall bring forward proof that there is a psychological technique which makes it possible to interpret dreams, and that if that procedure is employed, every dream reveals itself as a psychical structure which has a meaning and which can be inserted at an assignable point in the mental activities of waking life.

—Dr. Sigmund Freud, *The Interpretation of Dreams*

Introduction

Over a century ago, Dr. Sigmund Freud pioneered the idea of a meaningful association between our psychology and dreams. He perceived dreams as products of our mental activity and devised psychoanalytic methods to determine the nature of that activity. However insightful Dr. Freud may have been, his understanding of the relationship between dreams and the mind was limited by his science.

Dr. Freud's theories on the mechanisms of mental function were primarily influenced by classical science. Evidence of this influence is in his *Project for a Scientific Psychology*, first published as an appendix to his Wilhelm Fliess correspondence (circa 1895). In *Project*, Dr. Freud applied Newton's laws of motion to the physiological apparatus of the human nervous system. His theories involving our nervous system's properties of "inertia" would later become the basis for his theories on the conscious and unconscious processes of the mind.

Freud perceived the mind as a homogeneous structure composed of distinct psychical processes. He perceived dreams as manifestations of the mind's unconscious processes. In the opening pages to the first edition of his great work, *The Interpretation of Dreams*, Dr. Freud describes dreams as the "first member of a class of abnormal psychical phenomena of which further members, such as hysterical phobias, obsessions and delusions, are bound for practical reasons to be a matter of concern…"[1] His view of dreams as abnormal mental phenomena was based on his perception of a relationship between the unconscious state of brain function and the mind's unconscious nature, which he perceived as a bastion of mental disorder. That skewed perception of an association between unconsciousness and the nature of the mind's unconscious propensity continues to this day in nearly every order of psychological study. Relative to brain function, no current order of study has produced a clear consensus on the distinction of the mind. What is the mind?

From this point forward, let us regard the mind as an environment of cognitive activity, within the brain, arising from brain function. Our minds are a product of our functioning brains. Freud formed his theories on the nature of the mind in a vacuum of technology to study the functioning brain. In a paper he titled the *Neuro-Psychoses of Defense* (circa 1894), Freud acknowledged a void in his era's means to measure theoretical aspects of "mental function." Perhaps unknown to Freud, a door to that means opened in 1858 with a precursor to the electroencephalograph (EEG), a device currently used to record and study electrical activity within the brain.

The "mirror galvanometer" was patented in 1858 by Lord Kelvin (William Thomson, as he was privately known) and was capable of detecting microamperes of electrical currents. Dr. Richard Caton, a London physician in the late 1800s, was the first to apply this device to brain study. In 1875, Dr. Caton published findings of electrical signals on the exposed brain surfaces of various animals he studied using the galvanometer. Galvanic study of the human brain did not occur until after World War One.

By the end of World War One, scientists were using moving photographic paper to record the galvanic patterns of activity they observed in animal studies. This device, now an EEG, was first used in human studies by Dr. Hans Berger, an Austrian psychiatrist. He published his findings in a 1929 paper and subsequently went on to discover distinct patterns of brain-wave activity, which he called alpha and beta waves. Most notable to dream study was Dr. Berger's finding of a distinction in brain-wave patterns between the sedate (sleeping) and active (wakeful) brain. Intrigued by Dr. Berger's work, Dr. Alfred Lee Loomis, along with colleagues E. Newton Harvey and Garret A. Hobart, discovered a correlation between the depth of sleep and five well-defined and rhythmic variations in the electrical output of the sleeping brain. In a 1935 *Science* publication, they became the first scientists to identify and describe these distinct variations. Classifying each variation by depth alphabetically from *A* to *E*, Dr. Loomis was also the first to describe the specific characteristics of the electroencephalographic patterns we now associate with non-REM sleep. In the science of dreaming, the next notable step came with recognition of its physiological signs.

Chicago researchers Eugene Aserinsky and Nathaniel Kleitman, in 1953, described a relationship they observed between the intervals of rapid eye movement (REM) during sleep and the incidences of dreaming their research participants reported. When aroused during REM sleep, participants reported more incidences of dreaming than in any other sleep state the researchers observed. This association of REM with dreaming, along with the discovery of synchronous events involving heart rate and breathing, effectively gave dream research the distinctive physiological indicators required to establish the onset of dreaming in the sleeping brain. These indicators also gave dream research a basis from which to begin the neurological evaluation of the distinction between the conscious brain and the dreaming brain.

In 1959, Dr. Michel Jouvet of Claude Bernard University in Lyon, France recognized REM sleep as a distinct state of existence he termed "paradoxical sleep." Dr. Jouvet considered REM a paradox of sleep, because the brain's electrical activity during REM sleep was comparable to that of a conscious brain. His observation was significant in establishing dreaming as a type of wakefulness in the sleeping brain. Initially, Jouvet found the only determinable distinction between the conscious and the dreaming brain was the near-physical paralysis REM sleep seemed to cause. Interestingly, non-REM (NREM) sleep and true wakefulness do not involve movement inhibition. In later years, as our technology evolved, functional images of the dreaming brain would provide more information with detail and sophistication.

During a late-1980s metabolic study of the dreaming brain, using positron emission tomography (PET), Dr. Louis A. Gottschalk and his team of researchers at the University of California in Irvine found that some dreams can evoke regions of the brain associated with cognition, reasoning, and short-term memory. PET scans of the brain detect the short-term radioisotopes introduced in the brain via ingested glucose. These isotopes localize in active brain tissue through blood flow. Although this and similar technology have enhanced our neurological perspective of dreaming, they have not substantially advanced our unanimity on the psychological significance of dreams.

Most psychologists view dreams as meaningful tools in the diagnosis and treatment of mental disorder. In separate research, psychologists Paul Tholey and Stephen LaBerge have uncovered evidence supporting the therapeutic affects of a type of dreaming Tholey called *klartraume* (lucid dreams). However, some researchers and psychologists view dreams as merely meaningless mental byproducts of random cortical stimulation arising from internal biological processes.

In a September 1994 *Omni Magazine* article on lucid dreaming, Francis Crick, a discoverer of the DNA double helix, is mentioned as having speculated on dreaming as a process the brain uses to prevent data overload by eliminating "spurious memories." Psychologist Bill Domhoff of the University of California in Santa Cruz says he is "unimpressed with any evidence that dreams have a function or a purpose." He has done a statistical analysis on dream imagery and concludes dreams to be "an accidental byproduct" of evolution (*Discover Magazine* [2002]: 23[03]). So what is the answer? Are dreams truly meaningful or just random mental phenomena of no useful significance?

Whatever the intent of dreaming, it is not revealed by the psychological or neurological evidence alone. Discovering their precise purpose requires a merger of all available evidence. Psychology, as it relates to the processes and products of mental activity, is empirically impossible without an underlying neurological structure as its progenitor. The neurological evidence this book reveals and explores over several chapters shows that dreams, as probable psychological products, are not possible without the neurological structure we have evolved to support dreaming. We are incapable of any action, psychological or otherwise, without the intricate neural network and function of our central nervous system. This neurological perspective of dreaming is the basis for all the implications of dreams you will explore and discover through the *Neuropsychology of the Dreaming Brain*.

About ten days ago, I retired very late. I had been up waiting for important dispatches from the front. I could not have been long in bed when I fell into a slumber, for I was weary. I soon began to dream. There seemed to be a death-like stillness about me. Then I heard subdued sobs, as if a number of people were weeping. I thought I left my bed and wandered downstairs. There the silence was broken by the same pitiful sobbing, but the mourners were invisible. I went from room to room; no living person was in sight, but the same mournful sounds of distress met me as I passed along. I saw light in all the rooms; every object was familiar to me; but where were all the people who were grieving as if their hearts would break? I was puzzled and alarmed. What could be the meaning of all this? Determined to find the cause of a state of things so mysterious and so shocking, I kept on until I arrived at the East Room which I entered. There I met with a sickening surprise. Before me was a catafalque, on which rested a corpse wrapped in funeral vestments. Around it were stationed soldiers who were acting as guards; and there was a throng of people, gazing mournfully upon the corpse, whose face was covered, others weeping pitifully. "Who is dead in the White House? I demanded of one of the soldiers, "The President," was his answer; "he was killed by an assassin." Then came a loud burst of grief from the crowd, which woke me from my dream. I slept no more that night; and although it was only a dream, I have been strangely annoyed by it ever since.

—Abraham Lincoln, three days before his assassination, as told to Ward Hill Lamon

CHAPTER I: Meaning

Are dreams meaningful? In the minds of many, recounts like Mr. Lamon's have engendered little doubt. For many, dreams are a profound and unwavering source of insight. However, others remain skeptical and discount dream experiences like Lincoln's as purely coincidental. Obviously, coincidence is not reliable evidence of a meaningful association between dreams and reality. Reliable evidence is an essential component of the foundation upon which we seek to build our perspective of dreams and dreaming. Empirical evidence is better.

Information

Empirically, dreams are information. They are visual, oral, aural, olfactory, and tactile information about something a dreamer believes he or she experienced before waking from sleep. As Dr. Gottschalk's and other imaging studies have confirmed, the dreaming brain appears to accesses some of the same neurological structures and functions the conscious brain requires to interpret the physical world. If this brain activity is any indication, then dream imagery is clearly information about the influences the brain believes it experienced during sleep. Although this perspective of dreams as information may seem valid, it does not necessarily suggest that the information dreams provide is meaningful or useful.

Meaning

Whether the information dreams reveal is useful will be discussed in later chapters. As to whether it is meaningful, we need only define the nature of "meaning" and examine dreams in light of that definition. *Merriam-Webster's Dictionary* defines meaning as "what is intended to be or actually is expressed or indicated." In the purest sense, by definition, our dreams are meaningful when we can express or describe their imagery substantively. Consider the following dream:

> *I was wearing blue (I don't know if they were aqua or blue topaz) earrings. They kept on falling out all night when I was at a party. But I kept on finding them, thank God. They were not gold. Then I finally took them off and put them in my purse. Then I saw two girls: one was Chinese with a periwinkle-blue Hawaiian necklace and the other one was black with a pink fuchsia Hawaiian necklace. Weird!*

Contrary to the dreamer's critique, this dream was not at all weird; it was a meaningful experience. She had a sense of self and a sense of her surroundings, and most importantly, she could describe these experiences. Her description shows her recognition and identification of the influences she experienced. This dream was meaningful to the dreamer because she was able to recognize and identify its content substantively. It is meaningful to us because we can understand and envision her experience through the description she gave. For example, her description of wearing earrings does not mean she wore no jewelry in her dream. If the dreamer meant what she said, we understand that meaning through the words she used to describe her experience.

*   *   *

Thus far, we have tried to show how dreams could be viewed as meaningful information. Our dreams are information in that their content informs us about experiences we believe we encountered while asleep. They are meaningful in the sense that we are able to recognize and identify their content. They are also meaningful to others to the extent we are able to render descriptions of them. However, this perception of dreams as meaningful information is insufficient evidence of their usefulness. Meaningful information is not necessarily useful information. So what use are dreams? What purpose or function does dreaming serve?

REFERENCE

Bower, B. "A Thoughtful Angle on Dreaming." *Science News* (1990): 137(22): 348.

Buchsbaum, M. S., Gillin, J. C., Wu, J., Hazlett, E., Sicotte, N., Dupont, R. M., and Bunney, W. E., Jr. "Regional Cerebral Glucose Metabolic Rate in Human Sleep Assessed by Positron Emission Tomography." *Life Sci* (1989): 45(15): 1349–56.

Gottschalk, L. A., Buchsbaum, M. S., Gillin, J. C., Wu, J. C., Reynolds, C. A., Herrera, D. B. "Anxiety Levels in Dreams: Relation to Localized Cerebral Glucose Metabolic Rate." *Brain Res.* (1991): 538(1): 107–10.

Hong, C. C., Gillin, J. C., Dow, B. M., Wu, J., Buchsbaum, M. S. "Localized and lateralized cerebral glucose metabolism associated with eye movements during REM sleep and wakefulness: a positron emission tomography (PET) study." *Sleep* (1995): 8(7): 570–80.

These grand personages who set out to discover the great truth and never quite find it, give me a pain...They can't find it because they are always looking in the wrong place.

—Galileo Galilee

CHAPTER II: Truth

Galileo, whom Albert Einstein called the father of modern physics, lived during an age when church doctrine decided "the great truth." He was a man of science whose progressive observations on the nature of the cosmos stifled under his era's myopic adherence to religious edicts. Something like this could be said about current attitudes about the nature of dreams and dreaming. Among mind scientists, "the great truth" on the psychological nature of dreams was decided in the last century by Sigmund Freud and Carl Jung. The ideas of these learned men, particularly Jung's, have inspired levels of devotion reaching almost religious proportions.

Sigmund Freud

Time Magazine, in March 1999, listed Dr. Sigmund Freud among the twentieth century's one hundred most influential people, saying, "He opened a window on the unconscious...and changed the way we view ourselves." Although Freud began his career in traditional medicine, maladies of the mind became his all-consuming passion. His descriptions of the mind—its attributes and ailments—permeate our language and our psyche.

In the past century, Freud gave us a description of an instinctual part of the mind he called the id. He also gave us the term "ego" for the mental distinction he associated with our conscious sense of self. Freud associated our sexual idiosyncrasies with penis envy, castration anxiety, and Oedipus and Electra complexes. One of Dr. Freud's most important contributions to our lexicon of mental attributes was his description of the unconscious mind. "Unconscious" was how he described an aspect of the mind he associated with repressed feelings, desires, and memories. When we evaluate the science and methods Freud pursued to arrive at the terms we now use to define our mental structure and nature, we get a sense of where he may have been looking for "the great truth."

Dr. Freud had an ardent interest in maladies of the mind. In 1895, he authored a paper with Josef Breuer, a physiologist, on their study of hysteria patients. Although their paper referenced some theoretical aspects of the neuro-physiology associated with the mental illnesses they studied, their perspective was limited by the available science and technology of their era. In the opening pages of this book, we briefly discussed how the limits to studying brain function in Freud's era may have influenced his perspective of the mind. While animal stud-ies could have given him insight into some basic levels of brain function, Freud did not have the investigatory technology of the kind we enjoy today. Like most psychologists since his day, Freud followed an outside-in approach to the mind and the underlying psychology of manifest behaviors.

Manifest behaviors are the actions of the mind evinced by our behaviors and experiences. Dr. Freud was a keen observer of manifest behaviors. His observa-tions included what his patients did and what they said. Freud devised a mode of therapies focusing on the inorganic causes of the behaviors he observed. Freud called his method psychoanalysis and used it to elicit behavioral responses which he would then analyze for causative factors. Freud's descriptions of our mental structure were predicated on his observations of aberrant behaviors—behaviors for which his patients sought treatment.

Essentially, Dr. Freud's grand revelations on our mental structure and nature were determined by his evaluations of the words and deeds of the mentally ill. His dream-work was merely an extension of his work with these patients. He sur-mised the nature of the mind and of dreaming from aberrant examples.

Freud derived his ideas of the unconscious mind from his observations of aberrant behaviors arising from causes his patients were unaware of before their treatment. Arising as dreaming does during the unconscious state of sleep, Dr. Freud probably perceived dreams initially as unconscious forms of manifest behavior and then constructed his elaborate theories around this perception. However, associating descriptions of the unconscious mind with the unconscious sleep state, as Freud obviously did, is like describing the earth's core by its surface eruptions. Unfortunately, this error of perception and this misinterpretation of mental processes have remained unchallenged in the years succeeding Freud. In later years, a challenge of another sort would come to Dr. Freud's ideas via his protégé, Dr. Carl Jung.

Carl Gustav Jung

At the beginning of their association, Dr. Jung held a deep admiration for Freud. Freud, nineteen years Jung's senior, saw Jung as his heir apparent. Extraordinarily close initially, the two men would later part company over their divergent views. Jung went on to expand what he perceived as Freud's narrow perception of the unconscious. His vision included a perspective of the unconscious as manifesting both personal and collective influences. Jung found his version of "the great truth" through his spiritual quest and (like Freud) behavioral observations—primarily his own mingled with those of his patients.

Jung's early years were shaped by the intensely religious influence of his family. His father, Johann Paul Achilles Jung, was a Protestant orthodox minister who maintained an extensive library in which Jung spent many hours reading during his youth. However, Jung's introduction to alternative religions came when he was four years old through his mother, Emilie Preiswerk Jung, who provided him with illustrated children's books on Hinduism and other religions. Near the age of twelve, a powerful dream experience with religious overtones profoundly influenced his sense of spiritual significance.

Jung dreamed he saw God seated upon a golden throne and defecating on a church whose cathedral dome was shattered by his holy issue. This first appearance of a spiritual entity in his dream led Jung to believe himself to be among God's chosen. Believing his dreams issued from a source of wisdom beyond himself, Jung would soon begin to make decisions on his life's direction according to the messages he believed his dreams delivered. Over the years, Jung increasingly sought spiritual insight through sources beyond the boundaries of his era's religious establishment. From mythology to metaphysics, Jung also explored subjects exceeding the limits of accepted science in his era. Jung spent nearly two years researching séances and mediums.

Dreams and dreaming were integral to his spiritual quest. Subsequently, Jung's pursuit, quantified by his dream experiences, led to his groundbreaking theory of archetypical dream imagery issuing from a collective unconscious source. Through his comparative, cross-cultural study of dreams (including his own), Jung came to believe in the existence of an independent unconscious source of collective wisdom that the sleeping mind can access through the dream state.

Dr. Jung's notion of a force or influence beyond the self, underlying the nature of the individual unconscious, is radically difference from Dr. Freud's view. Freud perceived the unconscious as the repressed state of libidinous energies that erupt into aberrant behaviors, including dreaming. If we accept Jung's view, our dreams are heaven-sent. If we reject Jung for Freud, dreams are emanations from our own personal hells. In the realm of public opinion, Dr. Jung's view of dreams and dreaming has captured the minds of a devout majority. His spiritual perspective and hopeful approach has elevated his dream theories to levels currently eclipsing Freud's in popular appeal.

"The Great Truth"

According to Galileo, "the great truth" cannot be found when it is sought in the wrong place. If we are seeking truth on the nature of dreams and dreaming, we will not find it through either Freud's or Jung's theories. They never found the truth of dreaming, because they were not looking in the right places.

Dr. Freud's misstep in his search for truth came with his reliance on aberrant examples of the mind to define its structure and, by extension, the nature of dreams. His theories were based on his study of mentally ill patients. He perceived a relationship between the wakeful and dream states of these patients and interpreted all dreams according to his assessments of this relationship. Insight derived from imperfect examples is invariably representative of those imperfections. The insight Freud derived from imperfect mental examples defines his perception of those mental imperfections, not the mind in general. Our mental structure and the nature of our dreams are not defined by our mental imperfections, nor are they defined, as Jung clearly concluded, by our spirituality.

In *Life of Jung*, Ronald Hayman writes, "What the religious man calls God, [Jung] said, is what the scientific intellect calls the collective unconscious." Jung clearly disguised his spiritual idealism as science, saying (according to Hayman), "Man's vital energy or libido is the divine pneuma all right, and it was this conviction which it was my secret purpose to bring into the vicinity of my colleagues' understanding." Although Jung's spiritualism may not seem to be sufficient cause to invalidate his theories, he, like Freud, went looking in the wrong place for the true nature of dreams.

*   *   *

Our path to the great truth on the nature of dreams is lit by the following passage from the opening pages of this book: "Psychology, as it relates to the processes and products of mental activity, is empirically impossible without an underlying neurological structure as its progenitor...dreams, as probable psychological products, are not possible without the neurological structure we have evolved to support dreaming."

As psychiatrists, Freud and Jung merely concerned themselves with the psychological implications of dreaming. Freud focused on mental illness, while Jung pursued spirituality. In their many years of tireless devotion to deciphering various mental enigmas, neither Freud nor Jung seemed to thoroughly grasp the significance of neurophysiology to the enigma of dream production. Psychology references our mental dynamics, and dreaming is a dynamic process of the mind. However, the mind is a product of brain function. The brain is a neurophysiological zenith. Any theory about the true nature and processes of the mind is incomplete and unreliable without a comprehensive neurophysiological foundation. Neither Freud's nor Jung's theories include such a thorough foundation. Therefore, in the following chapters we will examine the neurological structures constituting our mental processes, with special emphasis on those that generate dreaming.

REFERENCE

Freud, S., Brill, A. A. *The Interpretation of Dreams*. London: Allen & Unwin, 1915; New York: Macmillan.

Gay, P. "Sigmund Freud." *Time Magazine* (1999): 153(12): 66–69.

Hayman, R. *A Life of Jung*. New York: Norton, 2002.

SUGGESTED READING

Freud, S. *Introductory Lectures on Psycho-analysis (Part III); General Theory of Neurosis (1916–1917)*. London: Hogarth Press, 1963.

Freud, S. and Sprott, W. J. H. *New Introductory Lectures on Psycho-analysis*. London: Hogarth Press, 1931.

Freud, S. and Strachey, J. *The Ego and the Id*. New York: Norton, 1961.

Freud, S. and Strachey, J. *The Standard Edition of the Complete Psychological Works of Sigmund Freud*. London: Hogarth Press, 1986.

Hull, R. F. C. *C. G. Jung: Dreams*. Princeton: Princeton University Press, 1974.

Jung, C. G. and Hull, R. F. C. *The Archetypes and the Collective Unconscious*. Princeton: Princeton University Press, 1968.

Storr, A. *The Essential Jung: Selected Writings*. Princeton: Princeton University Press, 1983.

Ulanov, A. B. *Religion and the Spiritual in Carl Jung*. New York: Paulist Press, 1999.

White, A. D. *A History of the Warfare of Science with Theology in Christendom.* New York: Appleton, 1898. (Chapter III, Astronomy, describes the religious war on Galileo.)

It was just a brain—the brain that dreamed a plastic fourth dimension, that banished the ether, that released the pins binding us to absolute space and time, that refused to believe God played dice, that finally declared itself "satisfied with the mystery of life's eternity and with knowledge, a sense, of the marvelous structure of existence."

—James Gleick's tribute to Albert Einstein's brain in a *Time Magazine* article on the greatest minds of the twentieth century

CHAPTER III: Foundation

In the human body, no single organ is more vital to bodily function and quality of life than the brain. It sits atop our central nervous system (CNS), which also includes the spinal cord. The brain is the pinnacle of neurological structure and development. It regulates our physical systems and the mental processes it generates interprets our experiences and individuality. The thoughts, emotions, and dreams we experience are products of brain function. The foundation of brain function is perception.

Perception

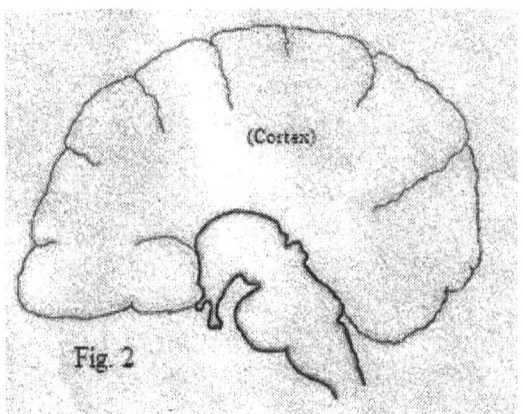

Fig. 2

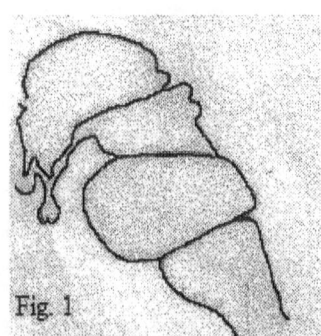

Fig. 1

Throughout this book, you will find different interpretations for several terms and processes traditionally used to describe attributes of mind, brain, and human psychology. "Mind," for example, is defined in this book as the environment of cognitive activity that brain function creates within the brain's structure. The primary initiate of brain function is perception; therefore, the primary initiate of the mind is perception. Perception, as interpreted here, is the detection of influence. It is the moment when the brain senses the impact of something it has experienced.

The brain perceives experience as source-encoded information, which it receives through an extensive and specialized system of internal and external sensory receptors and nerves. In the head, a network of receptors and twelve cranial nerves delivers visual, oral, aural, and olfactory sensory information to the brain through a substructure between the forebrain and the spinal cord called the brainstem (Fig. 1–2). An array of peripheral receptors and nerves in the body, dubbed the somatosensory system, conveys body sensory information such as position, movement, pain, temperature, and touch to the forebrain through the brainstem via the spinal cord. The influences these connections detect initiate those processes of brain function leading to the mental and physical distinctions upon which our consciousness and behavioral responses rely.

Physical Experience

Our ability to quantify the distinct nature of our physical experiences is a product of the information our brains receive about those experiences through their sensory systems. Anything experienced through the physical senses is distinguished by the brain as something it encountered in physical reality. Visual input, for example, stimulates a series of rods and cones in the eye called photoreceptors. Sensory impulses from these receptors travel along the optic nerve (cranial nerve II), which leads to the lateral geniculate nucleus of the thalamus in the brainstem. From the brainstem, these impulses primarily enter the occipital lobe of the cortex, where their visual information is assessed and distributed to other brain areas. In this example, sensory input from the eye is quantified in the brain as visual information originating from a physical source. However, not all information that the brain receives comes from physical sources.

Influence Impact

Nothing happens in the brain that is not a product of some neurological influence. Its behavior—the activity in which the brain engages—is a result of something it has experienced neurologically. Although physical experience is a primary source of neurological activity, the brain routinely engages in activities that do not appear to be a direct result of physicality. Dreaming is an example of such an activity.

Afferent Information

The dreaming brain, as Jouvet initially discovered, is virtually indistinguishable from the conscious brain. Our dream experiences appear to possess all the hallmarks of physical experience, with one significant exception: they are not physical experiences. Although every conceivable and inconceivable experience in physical reality can and does occur in dreams, they are not physical experiences. Physical experience is encoded by the afferent processes of our neurological structure. "Afferent" is a term which describes the neurological direction information travels into the brain from sensory sources.

Our brains perceive experiences as occurring in the physical world whenever our unencumbered senses deliver that information. The information our brain appears to perceive while dreaming is clearly not a product of the brain's direct contact with sources in the physical world. For example, dreaming about consuming a delicious red apple is not a result of actually having such contact with an apple while asleep. In this scenario, the brain is receiving information about eating an apple, when in reality the action is clearly not occurring. This paradoxical experience suggests that the information our brains perceive while dreaming originates from sources other than those our brains detect through our physical senses.

In separate experiments transecting the cortex from all other structures of the brain, Jouvet and Jaime R. Villablanca found that the cortex sustained a continuous state of slow-wave activity throughout the survival period of test animals. "Slow waves" denote the level of electrical activity, as measured by electroencephalogram, in the brain when it is not aroused, awake, or dreaming. Jouvet and Villablanca's results, important to all brain research, show that cortical activity does not occur independently of the cortex's substructures. While the cortex produces dreaming, it does not perform this function spontaneously or without subcortical connections.

In other experiments involving forebrain/midbrain border transection, the isolated forebrain resumed spontaneous electrical activity suggestive of arousal eight days after surgery. The forebrain includes the cortex and subcortical structures and is one of three archaic designations for the divisions of the brain. The other two are the midbrain and the hindbrain. The finding of resumed electrical activity in the forebrain after transection denotes the significance of cortical substructure to activity in the cortex.

All activity in the brain is a response to the information it receives. The imagery we experience while dreaming suggests that our brains are responding to information they are receiving. Without exception, all information arriving in the brain does so through its substructure, the brainstem. The brain activity constituting our dream experiences is also a result of information arriving through this important substructure.

We know that our dreams are not directly reflective of the information flowing from external sensory sources during sleep. A dream of eating apples when one is actually asleep in bed, for example, is not derived from information flowing from one's external physical experience. This suggests that our dreams are reflective of information flowing from internal sources. Since dreaming is a response to information and all information flows through the brainstem, our dreams must be reflective of information flowing from the brainstem without direct contributions from our physical senses.

Mental Experience

The role of the brainstem in the production of sleep and dreaming has been well researched, but not well understood by researchers. Nevertheless, the brain interprets information the brainstem generates while dreaming as something occurring within its structure—as mental experiences. Dreams are mental experiences without sensory contact with physical reality.

Although we may wake from dreams with memories suggesting real experiences in physical reality, our physical senses confirm otherwise when we become fully conscious. Our bodies' sensory systems encode the influences they detect as visual, oral, aural, olfactory, and tactile information. Because mental experiences originate from within our brain structures and not from our sensory receptors, the information our mental experiences produce is not encoded with the physical markers our senses provide. The brain's detection of this distinction is how we are able to determine whether our experiences are physical or mental ones. This distinction is particularly important to the efferent processes of the brain that are active and inactive during sleep and dreaming.

Efferent Information

If "afferent" describes the neurological path of information into the brain, "efferent" describes its outward path. Our internal and external organs and extremities receive information and instructions from our brain through a series of nerve connections leading away from the brain's structure. The behaviors and responses we manifest physically are products of these efferent nerve connections. During sleep and dreaming, our brains appear to suspend the connections associated with gross locomotion. Though we may seem to be doing much more in our dreams, our physical motions are limited to minor twitching during normal sleep. Why?

*   *   *

Why do our sleeping bodies remain virtually motionless when we dream? Since we are asking, why do our connections to our bodily senses appear to sever during sleep? The answers to these questions are, surprisingly, integral to the question of whether dream information is useful information. The path leading to these answers begins with a perspective on the evolution of sleep.

REFERENCE

Gleick, J. "Albert Einstein." *Time Magazine* (1999): 153(12): 74–78.

Kolb, B. and Whishaw, I. Q. *Fundamentals of Human Neuropsychology* (4th ed.). New York: Worth, 2000.

Jouvet, M. "Neurophysiology of the States of Sleep." *Physiological Reviews* (1967): 47(2): 117–177.

Jouvet, M. and Jouvet, D. "A Study of the Neurophysiological Mechanisms of Dreaming." *Electroenceph Clin Neurophysiol.* (1963): Suppl. 24.

Jouvet, M., Michel, F., and Courjon, J. "Sur un Stade D'activité Électrique Cérébrale Rapide au Cours du Sommeil Physiologique." *CR Soc Biol.* (1959): 153: 1024–1028.

Lamberg, L. "'53 REM Discovery Launched Study of Sleep Disorders, Treatment." *Psychiatric News* (2004): 39(1): 22–25.

Nolte, J. *The Human Brain: An Introduction to Its Functional Anatomy* (4th ed.). St. Louis: Mosby, 2002.

Villablanca, J. R. "Counterpointing the Functional Role of the Forebrain and of the Brainstem in the Control of the Sleep-Waking System." *J Sleep Res.* (2004): 13(3): 179–208.

I have now recapitulated the facts and considerations which have thoroughly convinced me that species have been modified, during a long course of descent. This has been effected chiefly through the natural selection of numerous successive, slight, favourable variations; aided in an important manner by the inherited effects of the use and disuse of parts; and in an unimportant manner, that is in relation to adaptive structures, whether past or present, by the direct action of external conditions, and by variations which seem to us in our ignorance to arise spontaneously.

—Charles Darwin, *The Origin of Species*

CHAPTER IV: Evolution

If you are among the many people who consider evolution to be more theory than fact, you will probably not accept some truths about the nature of dreams and dreaming. However, there is sufficient evidence supporting evolution. Researchers at the Digital Evolution Laboratory at Michigan State University in East Lansing have demonstrated evolution's impact on life through the breeding of digital organisms. With properties mimicking DNA, these organisms have allowed researchers to test and observe evolution through the effects on species development of a process Darwin called natural selection.

Natural Selection

Under natural selection, a species survives by developing attributes favoring its reproduction and survival. Through this process, a species can evolve from a simple organism into a more robust and adaptive life form. The human brain is a product of millions of years of evolution. It evolved from a simple colony of eukaryotes into an intricate network of neurological structures whose functions manifest the complex and distinctive behaviors we require to survive. Dreaming is a byproduct of the survival behavior we call sleep. It is considered a byproduct of sleep because, excluding physiological abnormalities, dreaming only occurs when we sleep. Considering what must have been incredibly harsh and hostile living conditions, our primal ancestors likely would not have evolved dreaming progeny without some advantage that sleep provides to the survival of our species.

Sleep *vs.* Survival

A behavioral evolution that clearly places a species in periodic states of apparent physical vulnerability seems incompatible with the goal of survival; however, this is exactly the general effect of sleep. Infancy and illness aside, humans are never more vulnerable than when they are asleep. Sleeping animals like us prevail today because sleep, at some point in prehistory, favored species survival. We sleep because it gave humanity's progenitors some advantage over predators, competing species, and adverse environmental conditions. When we examine sleep studies on contemporary animals, including humans, we find similar physiological effects, suggesting a shared survival strategy and advantage among early animals. Research on the effects of sleep among contemporary species, combined with the archeological record of life on Earth across several million years, offers a glimpse of the pivotal and primary advantage leading to the propagation of sleep.

Sleep Research Evolution

The neurological distinction of sleep from wakefulness was initially recognized by Dr. Hans Berger in the late 1920s through his study of electrical activity in the human brain. In 1935, Dr. Alfred Loomis and his colleagues further defined this distinction with their discovery of five rhythmic variations in the brain's electrical activity during sleep. Dr. William Dement (coupled with Dr. Aserinsky and Dr. Kleitman's discovery of rapid eye movement, or REM) further defined the human sleep cycle as consisting of four stages of NREM sleep followed by a stage of REM sleep that in 1959 Jouvet called "paradoxical sleep." The technological techniques and scoring of human sleep stages was standardized for research in 1968 through the work of Dr. Allan Rechtschaffen and Dr. Anthony Kales. In subsequent years, this research (which has also included nonhuman subjects) has provided a vast amount of information about the nature and effects of the various sleep stages.

S-sleep

In EEG studies, NREM sleep is characterized by four distinct stages of progressively synchronous, low-frequency waves. Researchers have called this quiet type of sleep "slow-wave sleep" or "S-sleep." Among contemporary mammals, S-sleep is characterized by a number of physiological effects. Significant for several reasons, S-sleep is our primary focus here, because the evidence in science points to it as the behavior from which dreaming evolved. Some physical effects of S-sleep include decreased respiration, reduced heart rate, and lower blood pressure. All of these are suggestive of the lower basal metabolic rate (BMR) of sleeping animals. BMR is the minimum caloric intake a resting animal requires to sustain life. The induction of S-sleep produces economy of motion and diminished physical perceptions and responses to stimuli. As a result, S-sleep reduces the demands upon the energy stores of a sleeping animal and decreases its metabolic rate to its lowest level. The physiological mechanisms controlling this aspect of sleep reside in the brainstem.

Brainstem

The brainstem is that part of brain structure situated between the forebrain and the spinal cord. In mammalian brains, it is composed of four segments: the myelencephalon (spinal brain), the metencephalon (across-brain), the mesencephalon (midbrain), and the diencephalon (between-brain). Although each segment contains structures that mediate important aspects of the sleep process, sleep production is coordinated by a layer of neurons between the thalamus and the hypothalamus in the diencephalon known as the ventrolateral preoptic nucleus. Aside from sleep, the brainstem's components regulate every aspect of vertebrate physiology and behavior through various neuronal connections that have evolved over several million years.

Cambrian Period

Second only to the spinal cord, the brainstem is the most primitive structure of the central nervous system in vertebrates. Scientists have found the earliest examples of brain and brainstem development among the fossilized endocasts of *haikouella lanceolata* (Fig. 3) from the Cambrian period of life on Earth, over 525 million years ago. An absence of fossil evidence among Precambrian animals

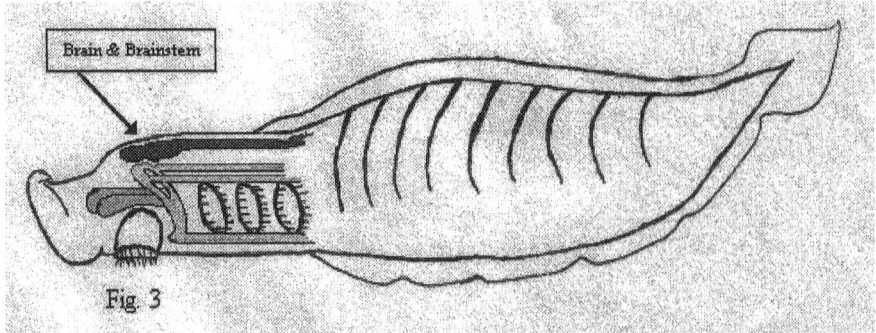

Fig. 3

(over 540 million years ago) suggests that the brainstem evolved during this crucial Cambrian period of species development.

The fossil record of the Cambrian period shows an explosive growth in the population and diversity of global life. This period is very often described as the Cambrian "explosion." Throughout our planetary history, increased population and species diversity have placed a premium on survival. A growing population must have adequate sources of food to sustain it. Coupled with increased diversity, the competition for food becomes more aggressive and predaceous as a population swells. Adapting to growing Cambrian populations would have required emerging species to develop survival strategies to sustain them as food sources dwindled and foraging became increasingly perilous.

Any Cambrian species that could suspend its demands for food through periods of hardship would have had a considerable advantage over those that could not. Among predaceous species, the suspension of appetite may have diminished the threat of their attacks on more rapidly reproducing prey species. This would have enhanced the availability and continued proliferation of significant food sources.

S-sleep Energy Conservation

There is evidence among contemporary animals showing that S-sleep reduces their demand for energy; therefore, their demand for sustenance during this sleep process is also reduced. S-sleep is regulated by a primitive brain structure (the brainstem) emerging during a period in prehistory (the Cambrian) when an effective strategy for enduring limited access to food sources was probably necessary to life. The Cambrian emergence of the brainstem (and the effect its S-sleep processes have on limiting energy needs) suggests that sleeping evolved as an effective means of regulating appetite, thereby conserving energy between cycles of feeding. The primary reason S-sleep characteristics persist among contemporary animals is to conserve energy.

D-sleep Energy Expenditure

Although S-sleep conserves energy, REM sleep appears to reverse this effect. In the late 1980s, Dr. Monte S. Buchsbaum and his colleagues at the University of California in Irvine studied the metabolic rate of glucose in human sleep. Glucose is the form in which our brains receive energy from the food we eat. Perhaps as expected, Dr. Buchsbaum's study revealed a marked decrease in the brain's overall level of glucose uptake during S-sleep. However, REM sleep produced significantly higher regional levels of glucose metabolism—higher in some brain regions than those observed during distinctly conscious states.

The EEG waveform pattern of the human brain in REM sleep is similar to that of wakefulness. This pattern is characterized by desynchronized waves of low amplitude and high frequency. Researchers refer to this desynchronized "wakeful" state of brain activity during REM sleep as "D-sleep." D-sleep negates the energy-conserving effects of S-sleep in the brain by increasing the brain's demand for energy. As a result, many sleep researchers discount energy conservation as a primary reason for sleep. However, those researchers have failed to fully uncover, consider, or comprehend a principal distinction posited by the evolution of D-sleep. (See **D-sleep Principle Distinction**.)

Decerebration

Sleep behavior arose as a survival strategy of Cambrian life-forms that had begun to develop simple brains and become more abundant and diversified. We know this behavior coincides with the evolution of the brainstem, because this is where we have found, in studies of animals and humans, sleep's neuronal mechanisms. When we examine these studies more closely, we find that the distinct physiological and neurological elements of sleep behavior evolved in stages corresponding to each level of the brainstem's evolution. Evidence of the first stage of sleep was found by Sir Charles S. Sherrington through his experiments with decerebrate animals.

Low-Decerebrate

Near the end of the nineteenth century, Sir Sherrington, who would later became a professor at Oxford and a Nobel laureate, researched the neural localization of the reflexive responses in cats through the successive removal of brain tissue descending through the brainstem to the spinal cord. He was able to localize the reflexive system associated with muscle tone in the brainstem's metencephalic region (Fig. 4). Animals whose brain tissues are removed or transected to this level are called low-decerebrate. Sherrington observed exaggerated stiffening in the musculature and posture of low-decerebrate cats; he called this "decerebrate rigidity." When left undisturbed, these animals lost their rigidity (tonicity) and collapsed into an atonic state. This cycle of tonicity and atonicity was observed in subsequent experiments by Dr. Jouvet, who in 1963 would describe the behavior as evidence of the "rhomencephalic phase of sleep."

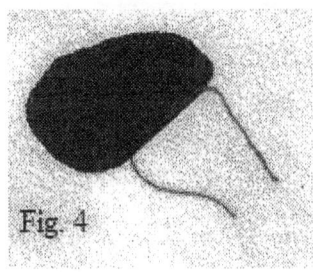

Fig. 4

Tonic and Atonic Sleep

The cycle of tonic and atonic muscle posture that Sherrington observed also manifests during normal sleep. The human sleep cycle consist of four stages of NREM followed by a single stage of REM throughout the progression of sleep. NREM sleep is accompanied by persistent muscle tone, while REM is not. Although low-decerebrate animals do not experience normal sleep, Jouvet viewed their tonic to atonic collapse as evidence of REM sleep behavior. His EMG (electromyogram) of the electrical activity in the musculature of these animals during atonia yielded comparable results to those of intact animals during normal REM sleep. However, his concurrent EEG studies of their brain activity only showed the distinctive spindle waveform patterns of NREM sleep. This finding of S-sleep brain activity with D-sleep muscle activity in low-decerebrate animals suggests the concurrent origins of S-sleep and atonia at the metencephalon level.

In all studies of decerebrate animals, none of the distinctive waveform patterns of brain activity associated with dreaming appear without the inclusion of diencephalic brain structures. Essentially, Jouvet's experiments with low-decerebrate animals showed that the muscle activity associated with D-sleep did not arise during the same period in brain evolution as the brain activity associated with D-sleep. In simpler terms, his experiments showed that the physical behavior we associate with sleep and dreaming appears to have evolved before the mental activity we associate with dreaming.

Muscle-Readiness Suspension

According to the evidence we have seen so far, S-sleep evolved during the metencephalic phase of brain development as a method to conserve energy. The metencephalon imposed energy conservation on animals through physical inactivity as a survival strategy. The animals that were most adept at surviving periods of diminished food resources were those that could effectively manage their metabolism through suspended activity.

A suspension of activity leading to the periodic loss of muscle tone decreases the energy requirement of those structures. Muscles require less oxygen and deplete fewer minerals when they are relaxed. With the ability to suspend activity in their muscles, primitive animals may have devoted their limited energy reserves to organs more vital to their survival during extended periods between feeding. This is precisely what we observe in present-day animals during the sleep-paralysis or atonic phase of D-sleep.

Energy Diversion

During the dreaming phase of sleep, we experience a complete loss of muscle tone and the devotion of more energy to the brain, heart, and lungs. We also experience what appears to be a loss of thermoregulation, but what is actually the internalization of thermal energy to further sustain and protect vital organs. In early animals, the internalization of energy reserves away from their musculature was a natural progression from a state of readiness to a state that preserved their vital systems between feeding cycles.

S-sleep to D-sleep

Compared to D-sleep, S-sleep is a more restful state of sleep. S-sleep decreases the energy demands of both brain and body. In human and animal studies, it is characterized by lowered brain activity, respiration, blood pressure, and heart rate. Also, S-sleep is uniquely distinguished by decreased but persistent muscle tone and the ability of the sleeper to quickly arouse from this state. During the

Cambrian era, S-sleep allowed animals to conserve energy through periods of physical inactivity and food privation by decreasing the energy demands of their evolving brains and bodies while maintaining a state of muscle readiness. When activity was required and food became available, they could quickly arouse to feed and replenish their energy stores. If an inactive or privation period persisted beyond their S-sleep endurance, these primitive animals would have required a survival strategy to extend that endurance until the restoration of activity and food resources. Extending the duration of sleep appears to be the overall effect of atonic sleep. In contemporary animals, Cirelli and Tononi has found that inactivity of the central noradrengeric system (locus ceruleus) during atonic sleep enhances protein synthesis in the brain.

Proto-sleep

The physiological and fossil evidence suggests that sleeping began as a survival behavior millions of years ago. In the beginning, the sleep/wake cycle of animals likely consisted of brief inactive (or partially inactive) periods followed by periods of more extensive activity. From the physiological evidence comparable contemporary species provide, we know early animals developed all the physical aspects of sleep behavior before developing the brain activity associated with dreaming; therefore, dreaming was not part of the early period of sleep evolution. This purely physical sleep, or proto-sleep, effectively imposed energy efficiency on evolving Cambrian life-forms by reducing their metabolisms when possible and increasing their metabolisms to sustain their vital organs when necessary. It was a successful survival strategy between cycles of feeding and during extended periods of food privation. However, proto-sleep would not have been as successful without the capacity to arouse from the state of inactivity it imposed.

Wakefulness

Wakefulness, regardless of sleep form, is essential to survival. The ability to arouse from sleep to obtain sustenance and respond to threats is necessary to the survival of all sleeping species presently in existence. Arousal from proto-sleep to feed or to fend off survival threats would also have been a necessity of Cambrian life. As a Cambrian species became more energy-efficient, it would not have needed to arouse from inactivity as frequently as less efficient animals. If this species was also a top predator, it could have extended its proto-sleep period even longer. However, if the species was prey, it would have had to remain more vigilant and spend less time in proto-sleep. The predaceousness of the Cambrian period is evident among the fossil remains from the Burgess Shales of Canada. Among those remains, archeologists have found trilobite fossils bearing the distinctive bite marks of a formidable extinct predator called *anomalocaris canadensis*.

S-sleep/D-sleep Summary

The evidence, in correlation with contemporary animal studies, show the brains of proto-sleep species evolving as their need for arousal to full wakeful activity diminished. Contemporary animals do not routinely arouse from S-sleep—the sleep associated with proto-sleep brain activity—to actively engage in physical experience and influence. Instead, they begin to dream. In relative terms, this might suggest that preexistent animals became more proficient survivalists and did not require frequent arousal as their brains grew and they became more intelligent. It is a good, but not necessarily valid, assumption.

The physiological evidence shows that dreaming activity in the brain evolved as part of sleep behavior during the diencephalic period of brainstem evolution. Below the diencephalon in representative species, we do not find the brain development associated with species intelligence. We do not find the gray matter configuration or function suggestive of thought and reason. Instead, what we find is the innervation associated with specific types of sensory perception.

Metencephalon/Tactile/Aural

In the mesencephalon of current animals, we find efferent nerve fibers associated with vision and chewing (cranial nerves III and IV). At the metencephalon level, we find afferent fibers associated with facial sensations, taste, and hearing (cranial nerves V, VII, and VIII). The appearance of facial and hearing afferents is particularly important to the evolution of sleep in primitive animals. The tactile sensory input of facial afferents meant that predators did not have to arouse to full activity unless prey or competition was detected. Hearing was important to sleep development in primitive prey, because it meant they could sense the approach of a predator by its sound; therefore, they did not have to arouse unnecessarily and expend precious energy reserves in order to secure their survival. Whether predator or prey, tactile and aural senses would have greatly enhanced a species' survival chances. (See **Cerebellum, Aural Sense, Tactile Sense.**)

D-sleep/Sight

At the D-sleep and diencephalic level of brain development, we find the entry of visual sensory information via cranial nerve II. Although visually receptive structures in the mesencephalon (superior colliculi, Fig. 16) suggest the dawn of sight at an earlier level, sight did not arise before the evolution of the diencephalon. In the human brain, the superior colliculi are anatomically out of position from their location when they first appeared. As the brain grew, these structures shifted posteriorly and inferiorly from their original place in the diencephalon region. This is why some mesencephalic EEG sleep studies show wakeful activity. Nevertheless, sight was perhaps the most important development in brain evolution. Visual perception meant that primitive animals could see whether the sensations or sounds arousing them from proto-sleep were worthy of a more active response. This suggests that primitive animals did not begin to extend S-sleep into D-sleep as they became more intelligent; they extended S-sleep into D-sleep as they became more sensorially perceptive.

Extended Inactivity

As the brains of preexistent species evolved, they became more perceptive and better at surviving. Armed with sensory abilities that extended their detection of prey, predators, and competition, these animals were able to extend their periods of inactivity and conserve energy after proto-sleep by arousing just enough to assess their sensory environments. This extended period of inactivity also might have been conducive to the repair of injuries suffered through conflict or mishap by diverting animals' energy reserves to tissue repair and regeneration instead of movement.

D-sleep Principle Distinction

The evidence shows D-sleep and atonia evolving during separate periods in brain development. Atonia evolved during the period when preexistent animals obtained tactile and aural senses, and D-sleep evolved when they obtained sight.

With sight, an animal was able to survey its environment with an economy of motion. After arousing from proto-sleep, primitive animals with sight did not have to become unnecessarily active when they had no pressing survival need. Unless they had a need to feed or to escape a threat, these animals likely reentered a proto-sleep state after each period of arousal. This arousal period after proto-sleep was a precursor to what we now experience as D-sleep, or dreaming. In reality, dreaming is not a type of sleep; all the evidence shows dreaming to be a type of wakefulness. The principle distinction overlooked by nearly every sleep and dream researcher since the inception of such work is that D-sleep is not sleep.

D-sleep Mesencephalic/Metencephalic Paradox

D-sleep is a misnomer; neurologically, dreaming is not a type of sleep. Excluding the appearance of a sawtooth pattern of waveforms detectable near the temporal lobe, the state the brain enters to dream is nearly indistinguishable by EEG from its conscious state. However, Jouvet's findings of rapid eye movement along with the spindles of S-sleep in high-decerebrate and low-decerebrate cats appear to contradict the wakeful origins of dreaming in the diencephalon.

Preparation Effect/REM

D-sleep is characterized by distinctive low-amplitude, high-frequency EEG waveforms in the brain. We do not find this pattern occurring during sleep before the diencephalic level of brain structure. At this level, we find the first appearance of visual sensory data entering the brain. The brain coordinates this sensory data with eye movement commands issued through its efferent oculomotor nerve fibers (cranial nerves III, IV, and VI) in the mesencephalon and metencephalon. These fibers are severed during the mesencephalic and metencephalic preparations for study. These preparations surgically sever the command hierarchy of the brain from the nerve fibers dedicated to that hierarchy in the brain's substructure. In a reversal of phantom-limb syndrome and akin to the spastic movements that acutely manifest in severed limbs after separation, the neurons of these severed motor fibers in the mesencephalon and metencephalon may continue to signal commands to the musculature of the eye and evoke movement. However, these commands would be random, weak, and masked by the ambient and more potent neural activity of an active mesencephalic/metencephalic brain. When neural activity in this brain diminishes, we see what Jouvet observed: eye movements that are slower and less frequent than normal REM. The REM Jouvet and others observed in animals without diencephalic brain structures was not evidence of D-sleep or dreaming; it was merely the breakthrough effect to the eye musculature of sympathetic signals from the severed oculomotor nerves embedded in the mesencephalon and metencephalon.

In the intact brain, REM is evidence of D-sleep or dreaming because of the dreaming brain's intact connection to the musculature of the eye. Any eye movements observed during sleep without this connection are not a product of dreaming or produced by the remaining structures of the brain. The severed nerves embedded in these remaining structures do not receive input from the surrounding tissue. If efferent nerve fibers were capable of receiving input from enveloping tissue, no command from the brain's hierarchy would reach the musculature of the body as intended. True REM suggests the directed neural activity of the dreaming brain.

Sleep to REM Evolution Summary

The evolutionary evidence tells us that sleep arose from our ancestral need to conserve energy. It also tells us that rather than a type of sleep, dreaming is a type of wakefulness. The repetitive cycle of sleep to dreaming that we presently experience during each period of slumber arose from our ancestral cycle of inactivity to arousal. We now know that REM evolved with the acquisition of sight at the diencephalic level of brain development. We learned that eye movement is a product of the wakeful behavior our ancestral species adapted to minimize energy depletion from gross movement. Finally, we have learned that atonic sleep evolved as a survival strategy to extend the endurance of inactivity between periods of feeding by redirecting energy to sustain vital bodily systems. In preexistent animals, this redirection of energy sustained their developing visual brains, which soon began to arouse during sleep to dream.

Diencephalon Wakeful Distinction

By looking at each level of brain development we have shown, we can track the evolutionary path our ancestral species traveled to reach the level of brain activity we associate with dreaming. At the metencephalon level, early animals acquired the behavioral and physiological characteristics of tonic and atonic sleep. Upon reaching the diencephalic (Fig. 5) level of brain development, these animals acquired sight and the mental (wakefulness) and physical (eye movement) characteristics indicative of dreaming. The acquisition of sight and the energy-conserving effect of muscle atony meant that our ancestral species could minimize energy expenditure in one respect while expending energy to remaining alert in another. A continuous state of alertness is distinctive of diencephalic animals.

Diencephalic Animals

In cats, dogs, and other animals with diencephalic brain preparations, researchers have observed profound states of hyperactivity and insomnia. Although the EEG and EMG at the mesencephalon level of these animals show results suggestive of tonic and atonic sleep, their intact diencephalons continuously register wakeful activity. So long as these animals are fed, their diencephalic activity remains in this hyper-alert state. Along with this alertness, the constituent structures of the diencephalon appear to contribute qualities integral to the nature of dreaming.

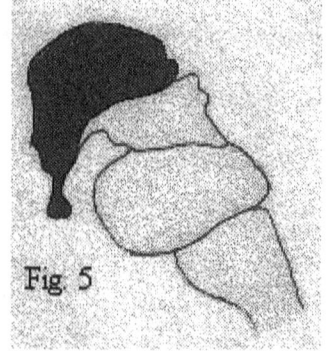

Fig. 5

Diencephalic Structures

The structures that make up the diencephalon are the hypothalamus (Fig. 6), the subthalamus, the thalamus (Fig. 7), and the epithalamus, which includes the pineal gland. Although researchers have not completely uncovered the behavioral intricacies these structures contribute, what they have found is quite significant.

Hypothalamus

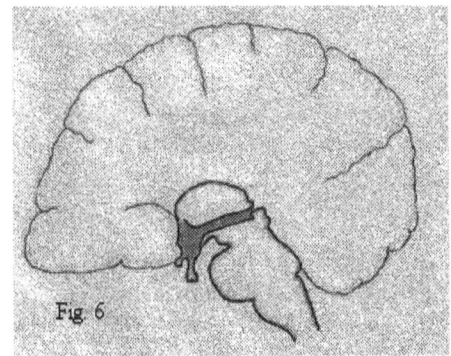

Fig 6

Some of the functional and behavior controls that the hypothalamus mediates are the autonomic nervous system and pituitary, as well as our hunger, sex, and emotional drives. With the evolutional development of this structure, we acquired the ability to autonomously regulate our respiratory, cardiovascular, gastrointestinal, and urogenital systems (homeostasis). During atonic sleep, the hypothalamus appears to lose some of its homeostatic ability: respiration becomes erratic, blood pressure rises, and body temperature falls. Nevertheless, this is also evidence of a functional hypothalamus and, as we shall see, its profound contribution to animal behavior and dream content.

Hypothalamus Emotion Research

In a 1925 issue of the *American Journal of Physiology*, Dr. Walter Bradford Cannon and Dr. Sidney William Britton described a "quasi-emotional" behavior in cats they had surgically prepared with intact diencephalic brains ascending through the hypothalamic level. The researchers called this behavior "sham rage." It was labeled as "sham" because this rage behavior could be summoned without an apparent cause. Cannon and Britton were able to elicit the behavioral characteristics of rage in these animals through hypothalamic stimulation. In later experiments, Dr. Philip Bard demonstrated the same results with just the posterior hypothalamus intact. These experiments, with this small section of the diencephalon intact, elicited a behavioral response associated with emotion. This was a momentous finding for behavioral and dream research, because it marks the stage in brain evolution where animals began to acquire a psychology.

Hypothalamus Psychology

Millions of years ago, our animal predecessors with hypothalamic brains began to develop what we now experience as affective conditions of the mind. They acquired the beginnings of emotions, suggesting the emergence of a psychology. Our erratic respiration and heart rate during atonic sleep are partly the physiological manifestations associated with the psychological responses the hypothalamus generates when its functions are released during atonia.

Although brain activity appears to slow during tonic sleep, Dr. Eric Nofzinger and his colleagues showed that cerebral blood flow to the hippocampus (Fig. 11a), the hypothalamus, and the metencephalic tegmentum (Fig. 13) remains relatively high compared to the overall decrease in the brain's blood flow before dream sleep. These findings suggest the continued function of these structures in maintaining the bodily systems they mediate. At the onset of atonic sleep, the metencephalon suspends its mediation of muscle readiness and releases the homeostatic functions of the hypothalamus it employs for quick arousal. The resulting impact on brain activity, caused by the suspension of muscle readiness during atonic sleep, affects the physical and psychological systems the hypothalamus mediates.

The Hypothalamus and Sexuality

The hypothalamus appears to mediate the sexual drive; this also supports the idea of an emerging psychology at its level of brain development in primitive animals. Sexuality suggests the emergence of socialization. Primitive, hypothalamic animals would have had to associate with their own kind to reproduce. Also, they would have had to develop socially connective behaviors to procure and maintain their reproductive associations.

During atonic states of sleep, when energy is diverted inward and away from our musculature, the hypothalamus is one of the brain structures this process feeds and releases. Among human males, we can observe an effect of hypothalamic arousal and its contribution to sexual function during atonic sleep. Penile erection is a trait among dreaming human males, from infant to adult, who exhibit normal physiology.

On the heels of psychological development, the next momentous step toward a dreaming brain came with the diencephalic evolution of the thalamus.

Thalamus Mind

In contemporary mammals, the thalamus has cortical relays for every sensory system and tissue of the body. It has visual (lateral geniculate nucleus), aural (medial geniculate nucleus), motor (ventral anterior and lateral nuclei), olfactory (dorsomedial nucleus), and somatosensory (ventral posterolateral and posteromedial nuclei) connections among several others leading to the cerebrum. In diencephalic animals, the

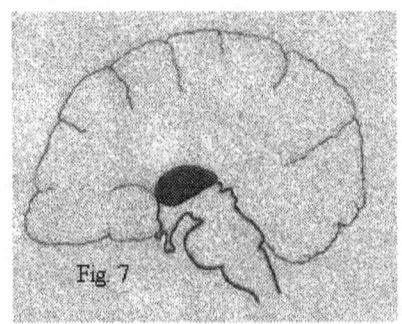

Fig. 7

thalamus would have been the destination of all sensory information. Thalamic evolution gave these animals an internal place to collectively sort and coordinate sensory information about their environments. Essentially, our ancestors with thalamic brains developed the ability to engage in the rudiments of thought; they developed a rudimentary mind.

Thalamus/Proto-brain

A mind, as we are learning, is an environment of cognitive activity within the brain, arising from brain function. When the thalamus appeared, our ancestors effectively developed a primitive brain capable of rudimentary thought. From its shape in present-day humans, we know that the thalamic brain looked very much like the modern human brain. The shape of the human thalamus has the characteristic left/right hemisphere and hemispheric adhesion (interthalamic adhesion, Fig. 8) that is typical of modern cortical structure. These proto-brains were the collection

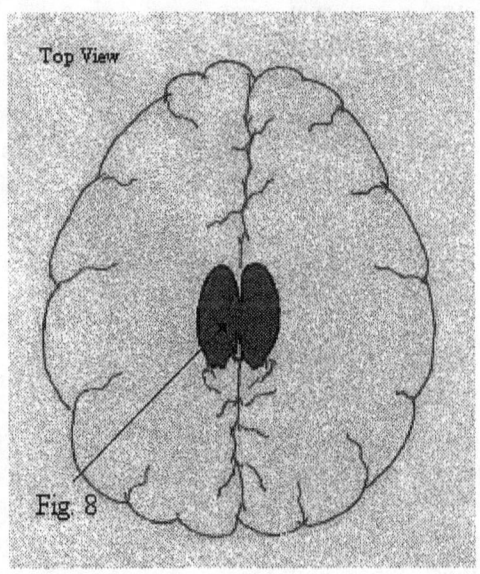

Top View

Fig. 8

centers for every sensation primal life-forms experienced. The hyper-alert behavior researchers have found among chronic diencephalic animals resides in this sensory-collection role of the thalamus.

EEG studies of diencephalic animals continuously register wakeful activity throughout their survival period, while substructures continue to cycle through tonic and atonic sleep. When the thalamus evolved, animals could centrally process sensory information and remain continuously alert through all states of sleep. Such behavior would have significantly enhanced their survival. However, this behavior would change considerably during the telencephalon level of brain evolution.

Cerebellum

The development of senses in early animals gave them new ways to gather information about their environments. At the metencephalon level of evolution, they acquired tactile and aural senses. At the diencephalon level, they acquired sight. Each level of sensory development brought new survival strategies. New senses meant new associative behaviors and the brain structures to accommodate those behaviors. In contemporary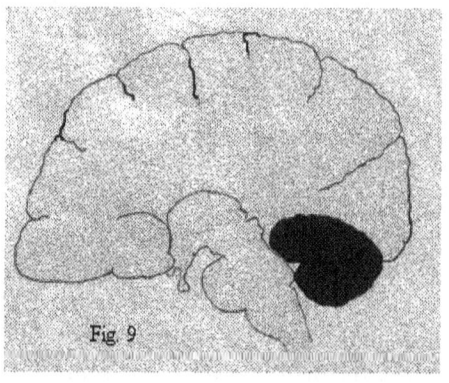

Fig. 9

humans, the cerebellum (Fig. 9) arises at the metencephalon level and is important to motion and balance. It evolved as our ancestral species acquired hearing. Although it arose prior to the telencephalic level of brain evolution, the cerebellum provided a quality precursor to what was to come.

Tactile Sense

In primitive animals, the tactile sense marked the beginning of motion. This type of sensory acquisition suggests that the behavior of these animals was influenced by physical sensations or contact. Sensations or contact possibly initiated associative physical responses, which might have included movements of withdrawal or attack. The ability to sense and grasp nutrients by touch, which also would have included taste, may have offered anchored species (akin to deep-water tube worms) sources of nourishment alternative to static resources; *e.g.,* ground nutrients and sunlight. Acquiring the sense of touch probably led to the sensing of tactile vibration, a precursor to sound detection. The deaf are sensitive to sound vibrations, which is a testament to the tactile origins of hearing.

Hearing

The acquisition of sound perception was an important milestone in species evolution, because it marked the beginning of directed locomotion. What we can gather about the mechanisms of hearing in primitive animals suggests that they were moving or orienting themselves either toward or away from specific sources of sound. For prey species, this movement would have allowed them to escape survival threats and forage for food. Instead of relying on chance encounters to obtain nourishment, foraging behavior would have allowed both prey and predators access to wider food sources. Among predators with sound perception, foraging might have involved orienting in a sweeping motion (a behavioral tactic with tactile origins) toward the sound of prey, and relying on touch for contact and capture. Standing in a fixed, upright position, a predator or prey animal with upper-body mobility could sweep its immediate surroundings or withdraw for protection at the first detection of a sound.

Balance

Foraging without sight probably would have required quick and balanced movements rather than precision movements. The wider a sightless forager's sweep of motion was, the more likely its location of nourishment would have been. The arrival of hearing at the metencephalon level likely influenced motion, requiring a better ability to balance. The cerebellum mediates balance in vertebrates and is evidence of the balance metencephalic animals required at their level of brain evolution. Upon the arrival of sight, balance was joined by precision through the evolution of the basal ganglia at the next and greatest level of our brain development, the telencephalon.

Telencephalon

The telencephalon is the final level of current brain development in humans. Its major structures include the basal ganglia (Fig. 10), the limbic system (Fig. 11), and the cortex (Fig. 12). Although some or all of these structures are present in the brains of other animals, the way their functions combine in the human brain has given our species dominion over all other forms of planetary life. The structures of the telencephalon have also given us a remarkable mental ability that other species with similar brain configurations possess: the ability to dream. Dreaming began with the evolution of the basal ganglia.

Basal Ganglia Research

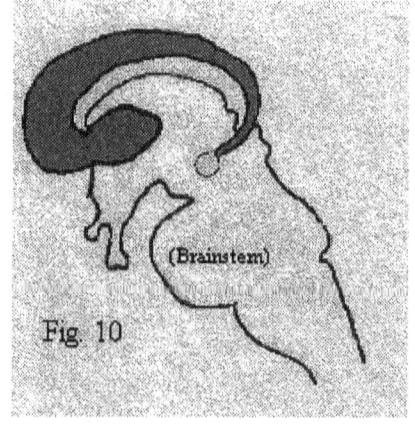

(Brainstem)

Fig. 10

In animal experiments with diencephalic preparations, researchers have observed behaviors suggestive of hyperactivity, deficits of coordination, and limited habituation to sensory stimulation. These were observed by Jouvet and Villablanca in cats, by Dr. H. J. Grill in his gustatory experiments with rats, and by Sir David Ferrier in monkeys. However, when these brain preparations included the section involving the basal ganglia, this behavior vanished conspicuously. In fact, decorticate animals—animals with basal ganglionic brain preparations—appear to behave as normally as animals with intact brains. With a little training, these animals eat normally, and they can engage in complex grooming and copulation behaviors. Most importantly, they appear to have normal sleep/wake cycles. Damage to or disease of the basal ganglia in the human brain can produce slow, uncontrolled tremors (athetosis) and spastic motions (hemiballismus). Sufferers may also experience bradykinesia (slow movement) or hypokinesia (decreased mobility). These disorders profoundly affect arm and leg movement. The conclusion scientists have drawn from the results of basal ganglionic research is that the basal ganglia are associated with movement. They are not far from the truth.

The current configuration of the basal ganglia has unexplained connections to the thalamus. Scientists studying these connections have been unable to clearly discern their purpose. Although science may know of no purpose for these structural links in the present day, they might have primal significance because of the quality these connections may have bestowed upon the developing senses and behaviors of early animals.

Coordination

Hearing triggered cerebellar development through a need for balance during the sound-initiated behaviors of early animals. When these animals acquired sight, they also acquired a need for precision of motion, as they needed to accurately target the objects they saw. With sight, foragers no longer required the sweeping motion of touch to sense food sources. The basal ganglia gave these animals the ability to steady themselves and position their limbs on specific targets. They could obtain objects they saw with direct, precise movements. The basal ganglia gave them better balance and coordination. This could explain why conditions like athetosis occur in humans when the basal ganglia are damaged. Athetosis is a derivative of Greek meaning "without position."

Basal Ganglia Distinction

By the time prehistoric animals reached the first stage of telencephalic evolution, they had acquired the ability to feel, taste, hear, and see. They had evolved cerebella for balance and basal ganglia for coordination. The basal ganglia likely dampened or mediated the excitatory effects of sensory experience on their thalamic brains. The resulting efficiency in movement may have given them more speed of motion and more steadiness during inactive wakefulness. This significant behavioral development might have made them more efficient foragers. It also would have enhanced the function of subsequent brain structures on the next step toward the dreaming brain.

Limbic System

At the thalamic level of brain evolution, animals began to combine multiple sources of sensory information about their environments through the unifying effect of visual perception. Before sight, behavior was instinctive or biologically reactive. They reacted to pain and pleasure received by touch, to nutritious and noxious substances received by taste, and to danger and calm discerned by sound. After acquiring sight, animals could combine what they felt, tasted, and heard with what they saw to initiate a behavioral response. As they became more visually dependent, their movements became more direct, coordinated, and swift. This dependency led to brain developments that gave our animal ancestors the ability to sustain tonic sleep after each stage of atonic sleep. The basal nucleus was one development and the others were the structures of the limbic system.

The limbic system (Figs. 11a and 11b) is a *C*-shaped body of structures in the lateral ventricle of the brain, surrounding the thalamus. For this treatise on dreaming, its relevant structures are the olfactory bulb, the hippocampus, and the amygdala. In several animal and human studies, these structures have been closely linked to emotions (amygdala), spatial learning (hippocampus), and memory.

Amygdala and Hippocampus Research

In 1957, Dr. Brenda Milner and a colleague noted the neurological significance of the hippocampus (Fig. 11a) to memory by observing the recent-memory deficits experienced by patients who had received surgical treatments for intractable epilepsy. These treatments involved the removal of the hippocampus and portions of the temporal lobe. Similar memory deficits related to learning were observed in primates by Dr. Elisabeth A. Murray and Dr. Mortimer Mishkin through their experiments in the early 1980s. Murray and Mishkin found the amygdala (Fig. 11b) to be more essential to learning than the hippocampus. They also noted that animals without amygdalae were more active, fearless, and disruptive than those with amygdalae. In experiments with decorticate animals that resulted in near-normal behavior, researchers did not excise this telencephalic structure. Animals with missing amygdalae were noted for their hyperactivity and lack of habituation. This suggests that the amygdala confers some calming quality upon behavior.

Memory

When early animals acquired sight, they also acquired the ability to identify what they felt, tasted, and heard. They could make visual distinctions about their environments and moderate their behavioral responses accordingly. As their dependence on visual distinctions grew, they gained the ability to recognize by sight the influences impacting their survival. This visual recognition was the beginning of memory.

Pain and Pleasure

Prey animals that recognized a distant predator could secure their survival at first sight. To have knowledge of impending peril from a distant animal, a prey animal would have required the ability to link the distinct visual markers associated with a predator to an effect on its physical well-being: fear. Fear is our most useful and instinctual emotion. It probably appeared the moment ancestral animals began to feel pain. Through the instinct of fear, animals secured their survival against physical threats. They also secured their survival through the instinct of pleasure. Taking nourishment and reproducing are instinctual behaviors driven by pleasure. In humans, eating and copulating affects the brain's pleasure centers. Fear, hunger, and sexual desire are all mediated by the hypothalamus. This structure receives afferents from the fornix of the hippocampus and from direct and indirect connections to the amygdala.

Taste

Until the arrival of visual perception, primitive animals identified influences in their environment through tactile perception. Taste is a tactile sense that evolved around the same time as touch during the myelencephalon period of brain development. It probably started as a process of molecular recognition upon contact at the cellular level of a feeding organism. Through taste, animals could identify the nutritional nature of the substances they felt. Animals with the ability to taste soon evolved into animals with the ability to detect the ambient molecules of food sources and other influences in their environments. The ability to detect and locate food sources by tasting ambient molecules can be seen today as it might have been in prehistory, by observing the sensory ability of contemporary reptiles. Some reptilian species can locate prey by the ambient taste of their prey's scent several miles away.

Taste and Sight

As ancient animals were beginning to associate their physical sensations with their visual perceptions, they were also beginning to associate their taste sensations with these perceptions. The myelencephalon arrival of taste before the diencephalon arrival of sight identifies taste as the more developed sense of the two. When sight joined with taste, animals were able to connect the ambient molecules they detected in their environments with the visual sources of those molecules. However, the adaptation of taste and feeding by the same orifice occluded the ambient detection of predators. Feeding animals could not detect predators through the orifices by which they fed.

Taste to Smell

We know taste evolved along with feeding orifices, because this is the most efficient configuration for the detection and quick consumption of nutrients. Primeval species with this configuration would have had a survival advantage over other species who could not immediately consume what they tasted. The ambient detection of prey, predators, or competition while these animals fed was also a survival advantage. The inability to detect these things while feeding likely led to the evolution of a separate orifice for such detection. This new orifice was the beginning of the olfactory sense.

Hippocampus

In mammals, olfactory data is gathered and delivered into the brain via the olfactory bulb (Fig. 11a) and the olfactory tract. The association of taste and scent with sight over several generations produced a brain structure that helped animals to mentally retain scent-oriented experiences. Although not currently defined in this way by science, the hippocampus coordinates our mental

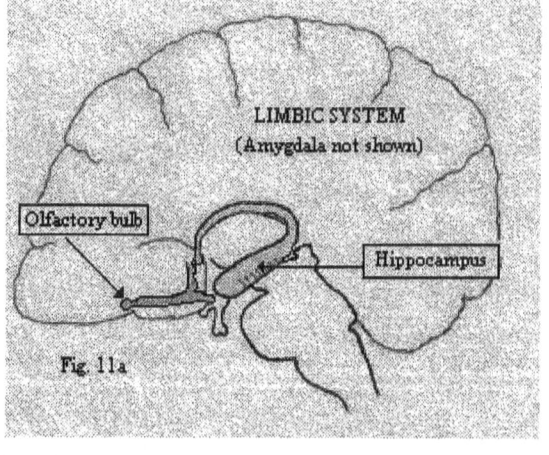

LIMBIC SYSTEM
(Amygdala not shown)

Olfactory bulb

Hippocampus

Fig. 11a

retention of scents. The structures of the human olfactory system have sensory pathways leading to the hippocampus, as well as to the amygdala and the hypothalamus. Armed with a hippocampus, an early animal would have been able to make behavioral choices according to the prior impact of specific scents on its survival instincts. The "spatial memory" effect found in hippocampus research is a result of scent-oriented perception, which is multidirectional. Lab experiments have shown that scent-dependent animals whose hippocampi have been destroyed have difficulty remembering their way around mazes.

Amygdala

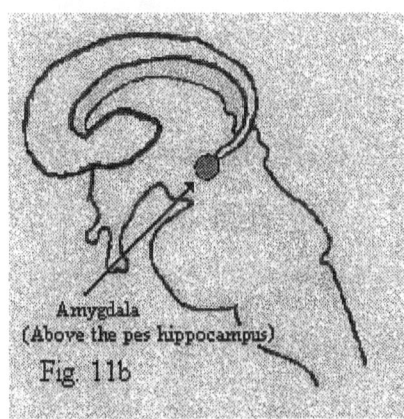

Amygdala
(Above the pes hippocampus)

Fig 11b

Coordinating multiple and repetitive sensory experiences produced, over countless years, a brain structure that helped animals to mentally retain the visceral effects of the experiences affecting their survival. As researchers like Murray and Mishkin have determined, the amygdala enhances the brain's learning faculty. This structure gave prehistoric animals the capacity to sustain the mental impact of pain and pleasure on their physical well-being. In contemporary animals, the amygdala has several afferents ending in the hypothalamus. Early animals with amygdalae were able to make behavioral choices viscerally; they could decide an immediate course of action by measuring the mental effects of their immediate experiences against the mental effects that persist from prior experience. Their viscerally distinctive behavior became what we call instinct.

Amygdala and Hippocampus Distinction

The principal distinction between the early amygdala and the hippocampus was that the amygdala gave early animals the capacity to preserve and recall the mental effects of painful and pleasurable experiences, while the hippocampus gave them a similar capacity with experiences related to scent. These structures are linked by sensory pathways in present-day animals.

Habitat Familiarity

Before sight, animals' behavior was driven by their instinctive and biological nature; *i.e.,* by pain and pleasure. When they acquired sight, animals could visually perceive the sources of pain and pleasure in their habitat. Over time and as their vision developed, they gained better coordination and speed. They became more proficient at identifying elements of their environment by mentally preserving the effects of those elements on their survival. Through their visual and olfactory acuity, coupled with the ability to remember, they could perceive peril or find food before physically encountering either one. The more readily an animal could perceive and identify things in its environment, the more familiar it became with its habitat and the better were its chances of survival.

Basal Ganglia and Limbic Distinction

The arrival of the basal ganglia brought coordination and steadiness. The emergence of the limbic system brought sustained habitat familiarity. In combination, the mental qualities these structures bestowed on early animals allowed them to maintain a continuous cycle of tonic and atonic sleep. Researchers have observed that test animals with these structures have the ability to learn; animals without basal ganglia and limbic systems do not learn from experience. These animals perceive all experiences as new. Their sensitivity to repetitive stimuli does not diminish. However, animals with basal ganglia and limbic systems do learn from experience. Early animals with these brain distinctions also learned from their experiences and became familiar with their habitats. They developed secure routines in which wakeful activity after atonic sleep was unnecessary. In an environment secured by their awareness through prior experience, they could sustain continuous cycles of tonic and atonic sleep until it was unsafe to do so. This placed our ancestral species on their final step toward dreaming as we know it today.

Cortex

Although sleep behavior began at the metencephalon level of brain evolution, the brain activity associated with dreaming did not emerge before the diencephalon level. All of the evidence shows dreaming to be a product of a wakeful and active brain. The EEG patterns associated with this distinction do not appear in the contemporary brain below the evolutionary level of visual perception. At this diencephalic level of perception, the brain

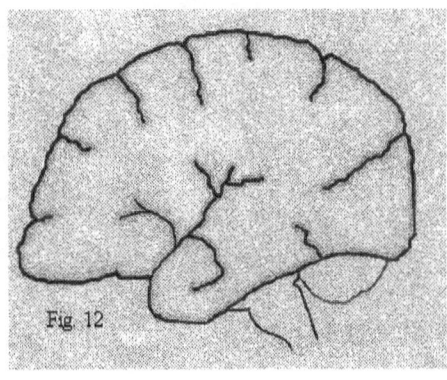

Fig. 12

began to behave proactively and evolved its first repository for sensory processing, the thalamus.

Sight, along with a thalamic brain, enabled behavioral responses independent of instinct. Animals became less reactive and more proactive as their visual recognition of survival-affecting influences awakened. This awakening enhanced their movements and spurred brain developments leading to better coordination and mobility. With increased mobility, their experiences grew and their brains evolved additional structures to help them remember experiences and the impact of those experiences on their survival. This mental retention of painful and pleasant effects helped them coordinate behaviors conducive to survival and catapulted them to our current level of brain development, the cortex (Fig. 12).

Anticipatory Behavior

When our animal ancestors began to retain painful and pleasant memories, they entered the telencephalon level of brain evolution. They had developed brains that were able to create a mental environment from which prior experiences could be recalled, enabling them to make behavioral choices that would lead to desired outcomes. This crafting of behavior to produce a desired outcome is called anticipatory behavior. Notably absent in decorticate animals, anticipation is the quality that cortical function refines and confers on behavior.

Decorticate Behavior

In studies of decorticate animals and congenitally decorticate humans, researchers have found few distinctions between their behavior and the behavior of those with intact brains. Decorticate animals appear to have normal sleep/wake cycles. They can stand, walk, and run. Even more amazing, they can engage in complex behaviors, such as copulation, and they learn almost as well as corticate animals of their species. The distinction conferred by the cortex is more clearly defined by subtle differences in the behavior of decorticate animals.

Subtle Distinction

Decorticate animals perform some acts of nesting, but do not build nests. Wishaw observed this in the behavior of rats; Overmier, Gallistel, and Rose saw it in the behavior of fish; and Miceli noted it in hamsters. Although they may carry food, they do not engage in hoarding or food-storing behavior. The subtle distinction between these types of behavior is that some nesting and food-related activities satisfy an immediate need or desire rather than an anticipated need or desire. In human terms, a decorticate man would not seek shelter or build it before the weather compelled him to do so. He would never conceive of planting crops. He would, however, fish and capture game, but only when the need arose. Decorticate animals do not anticipate what their needs or desires will be; they act only when needs or desires are evident.

Cortex and Wakefulness

The cortex gave early animals the ability to assess their potential needs and desires from memories of their experiences. Before this measure of brain development, they had begun to sleep and to experience sensory wakefulness whenever they entered atonic sleep. Sensory wakefulness was a survival strategy that emerged with the structures of the diencephalon and its visual sense. Before the emergence of sight, animals had developed a simple psychology. Animals with sight developed structures that produced a rudimentary mind. Through all of this development, sensory wakefulness continued.

Through sight, primitive animals were becoming more mobile and secure in their habitats. This produced new behaviors and new brain structures. Soon, animals were secure enough in their environments to enter sustained cycles of tonic and atonic sleep while their brains continued the wakeful strategy adapted earlier in its diencephalon evolutionary phase. This wakeful strategy during atonic sleep would now characterize the new behaviors, structures, and functions of the telencephalon.

Telencephalon/Cortical Distinction

The telencephalon, through its cortical evolution, gave our animal ancestors a unique advantage above all others. It gave them the ability to anticipate their needs and desires based on memories of the impact of prior experiences on their survival. When the newly evolved cortex began to wake during atonic sleep, it continued to assess and address the potential effects of influences in the animal's environment. In the present day, this process continues in all sleeping species in the cortical activity we call "dreaming." Dreaming is a mental process the brain engages during atonic sleep to assess influences of potential survival impact.

*   *   *

In concluding this chapter on the evolution of sleep and dreaming, we have made several distinctions. The function of sleep is to conserve energy. It emerged as a cycle of tonic and atonic activity of body musculature that was adapted to sustain survival through periods of diminished food resources. Atonic sleep is the more inactive and restful state of the muscles of the body, while tonic sleep is the more restful state of the brain and vital organs. We have also made the distinction that dreaming is not sleep; it is wakefulness. This wakeful activity of the brain during atonic sleep began at the stage in brain evolution when survival depended on sensory wakefulness during an animal's most vulnerable phase of physical inactivity. Finally, in its current incarnation, dreaming combines the functions of the diencephalon with the telencephalon during an arousal cycle that is initiated by metencephalic atonic sleep processes. This arousal creates an environment of cognitive activity within the brain that assesses the potential impact of affecting influences.

In the next chapter, we will more closely examine the activity the brain engages when dreaming and address the question of its usefulness.

REFERENCE

Aserinsky, E. and Kleitman, N. "Regularly Occurring Periods of Eye Motility, and Concomitant Phenomena, During Sleep." *Science* (1953): 118: 273–274.

Bard, P. "A Diencephalic Mechanism for the Expression of Rage with Special Reference to the Sympathetic Nervous System." *AJP* (1928): 84: 490–515.

Berger, H. "Über das Elektrenkephalogramm des Enschen." *Arch Psychiatr Nervenkr* (1929): 87: 527–570.

Büchel, C., Dolan, R. J., Armony, J. L., and Friston, K. J. "Amygdala-Hippocampal Involvement in Human Aversive Trace Conditioning Revealed through Event-Related Functional Magnetic Resonance Imaging." *The Journal of Neuroscience* (1991): 19(24): 10869–10876.

Buchsbaum, M. S., Hazlett, E. A., Wu, J., and Bunney, W. E., Jr. "Positron Emission Tomography with Deoxyglucose-F18 Imaging of Sleep." *Neuropsychopharmacology* (2001): 25(5): S50–6.

Buchsbaum, M. S., Gillin, J. C., Wu, J., Hazlett, E., Sicotte, N., Dupont, R. M., and Bunney, W. E., Jr. "Regional Cerebral Glucose Metabolic Rate in Human Sleep Assessed by Positron Emission Tomography." *Life Sci.* (1989): 45(15): 1349–56.

Cannon, W. B. and Britton, S. W. "Studies on the Conditions of Activity in Endocrine Glands, XV: Pseudoaffective Medulliadrenal Secretion." *Am J Physiol.* (1925): 72: 283–294.

Chen, J. Y., Huang, D. Y., and Li, C. W. "An Early Cambrian Craniate-like Chordate." *Nature* (1999): 402: 518–522.

Cirelli, C. and Tononi, G. "Locus Ceruleus Control of State-Dependent Gene Expression." *J Neurosci.* (2004): 24(23): 5410-9.

Conway, Morris S. "Burgess Shale Faunas and the Cambrian Explosion." *Science* (1989): 246(4928): 339–346.

Darwin, C. *The Origin of Species.* Chicago: Thompson & Thomas, 1872.

Dement, W. and Kleitman, N. "The Relation of Eye Movements during Sleep to Dream Activity: An Objective Method for the Study of Dreaming." *J Exp Psychol.* (1957): 53: 339–346.

Fellous, J. M. "The Neuromodulatory Basis of Emotion." *Neuroscientist* (1999): 5(5): 283–294.

Gallistel, C. R. *The Organization of Action: A New Synthesis.* Hillsdale: Lawrence, Elbaum, 1980.

Grill, H. J. and Norgren, R. "Neurological Tests and Behavioral Deficits in Chronic Thalamic and Chronic Decerebrate Rats." *Brain Res.* (1978): 143(2): 299–312.

Heiss, W. D., Pawlik, G., Herholz, K., Wagner, R., and Wienhard, K. "Regional Cerebral Glucose Metabolism in Man during Wakefulness, Sleep, and Dreaming." *Brain Res.* (1985): 18; 327(1–2): 362–6.

Jouvet, M. "Neurophysiology of the States of Sleep." *Physiological Reviews* (1967): 47(2): 117–177.

Jouvet, M. and Jouvet, D. "A Study of the Neurophysiological Mechanisms of Dreaming." Electroenceph *Clin Neurophysiol.* (1963): Supplement 24.

Kinnala, A., Suhonen-Polvi, H., Aarimaa, T., Kero, P., Korvenranta, H., Ruotsalainen, U., Bergman, J., Haaparanta, M., Solin, O., Nuutila, P., and Wegelius, U. "Cerebral Metabolic Rate for Glucose during the First Six Months of Life: An FDG Positron Emission Tomography Study." *Arch Dis Child Fetal Neonatal Ed.* (1996): 74(3): F153–7.

Kolb, B. and Whishaw, I. Q. *Fundamentals of Human Neuropsychology* (4th ed.). New York: Worth, 2000.

Lamberg, L. "'53 REM Discovery Launched Study of Sleep Disorders, Treatment." *Psychiatric News* (2004): 39(1): 22–25.

Loomis, A. L., Harvey, E., and Hobart, G.A. "Potential Rhythms of the Cerebral Cortex during Sleep." *Science* (1935): 81: 597–598.

Martin, C. R. and Marzec, M. L. "Sleep Scoring: 35 Years of Standardized Sleep Staging." *RT Magazine* (June 2003).

Mazzilotta, J. C., Phelps, M. E., Miller, J., and Kuhl, D.E. "Tomographic Mapping of Human Cerebral Metabolism: Normal Unstimulated State." *Neurology* (1981): 31(5): 503–16.

Miceli, M. O. and Malsbury, C. W. "Sagittal Knife Cuts in the Near and Far Lateral Preoptic Area-Hypothalamus Disrupt Maternal Behaviour in Female Hamsters." *Physiol Behav.* (1982): 28(5): 856–67.

Moore, J. W., Yeo, C. H., Oakley, D. A., and Russell, I. S. "Conditioned Inhibition of the Nictitating Membrane Response in Decorticate Rabbits." *Behav Brain Res.* (1980): 1(5): 397–409.

Murray, E. A. and Mishkin, M. "Severe Tactual as well as Visual Memory Deficits follows Combined Removal of Amygdala and Hippocampus in Monkeys." *J Neurosci.* (1984): 4(10): 2565–2580.

Netter, F. H. *Atlas of Human Anatomy* (3rd ed.). Teterboro: Icon, 2003.

Nofzinger, E. A., Buysse, D. J., Miewald, J. M., Meltzer, C. C., Price, J. C., Sembrat, R. C., Ombao, H., Reynolds, C. F., Monk, T. H., Hall, M., Kupfer, D. J., and Moore, R. Y. "Human Regional Cerebral Glucose Metabolism during Non-Rapid Eye Movement Sleep in Relation to Waking." *Brain* (2002): 125(5): 1105–15.

Nofzinger, E. A., Mintun, M. A., Wiseman, M., Kupfer, D. J., and Moore, R. Y. "Forebrain Activation in REM Sleep: An FDG PET Study." *Brain Res.* (1997): 3; 770(1–2): 192–201.

Nolte, J. *The Human Brain: An Introduction to Its Functional Anatomy* (4th ed.). St. Louis: Mosby, 2002.

Numan, M., Morrell, J. I., and Pfaff, D. W. "Anatomical Identification of Neurons in Selected Brain Regions Associated with Maternal Behavior Deficits Induced by Knife Cuts of the Lateral Hypothalamus in Rats. *J Comp Neuro.* (1985) 237(4): 552–564.

Oakely, D. A. "Performance of Decorticated Rats in a Two-Choice Visual Discrimination Apparatus." *Behav Brain Res.* (1981): 3(1): 55–69.

Overmier, J. B. and Hollis, K. L. "Fish in the Tank: Learning, Memory, and Integrated Behaviour," in R. P. Kesner and D. S. Olton (eds.), *Neurobiology of Comparative Cognition* (pp. 205–236). Hillsdale: Lawrence Erlbaum, 1990.

Rechtschaffen, A. and Kales, A. *A Manual of Standardized Technology Techniques and Scoring System for Sleep Stages of Human Subjects,* Bethesda: NIH, 1968.

Rose, J. D. "The Neurobehavioral Nature of Fishes and the Question of Awareness and Pain." *Reviews in Fisheries Science* (2002): 10(1): 1–38.

Saper, C. B., Chou, T. C., and Scammell, T. E. "The Sleep Switch: Hypothalamic Control of Sleep and Wakefulness." *Trends in Neuroscience* (2001): 24(12): 726–731.

Scoville, W. B. and Milner, B. "Loss of Recent Memory after Bilateral Hippocampal Lesions. *J Neuropsychiatry Clin Neurosci.* (1957): 12(1): 103–13.

Sherrington, S. C. "Decerebrate Rigidity and Reflex Co-ordination of Movements." *J Physiol.* (1898): 22: 319–332.

Shewmon, D. A., Holmes, G. L., and Byrne, P. A. "Consciousness in Congenitally Decorticate Children: Developmental Vegetative State As Self-Fulfilling Prophecy." *Dev Med Child Neurol.* (1990): 41(6): 364–74.

Shu, D. "A Paleontological Perspective of Vertebrate Origin." *Chinese Science Bulletin* (2003): 48(8): 725–735.

Siegel, A. and Brutus, M. "Neurosubstrates of Aggression and Rage in the Cat," in A. N. Epstein and A. R. Morrison (eds.), *Progress in Psychobiology and Physiological Psychology* (pp. 135–233). San Diego: Academic, 1990.

Siegel, J. M. "Mechanisms of Sleep Control." *Journal of Clinical Neurophysiology* (1990): 7(1): 49–65.

Skinner, D. M., Martin, G. M., Harley, C., Kolb, B., Pridgar, A., Bechara, A., and Van der Kooy, D. "Acquisition of Conditional Discriminations in Hippocampal Lesioned and Decorticated Rats: Evidence for Learning That Is Separate from Both Simple Classical Conditioning and Configural Learning." *Behav Neurosci.* (1994): 108(5): 911–26.

Sutherland, R. J., McDonald, R. J., Hill, C. R., and Rudy, J. W. "Damage to the Hippocampal Formation in Rats Selectively Impairs the Ability to Learn Cue Relationships." *Behav Neural Biol.* (1989): 52(3): 331–56. Erratum in *Behav Neural Biol.* (1990): 54(2): 211–2.

Tyler, K. L. and Malessa, R. "The Goltz–Ferrier Debates and the Triumph of Cerebral Localizationalist Theory." *Neurology* (2000): 55: 1015–1024.

Whishaw, I. Q. "The Decorticate Rat," in B. Kolb and R. C. Tees (eds.), *The Cerebral Cortex of the Rat.* Cambridge: MIT Press, 1990.

Whishaw, I. Q. and Kolb, B. "Decortication Abolishes Place but Not Cue Learning in Rats." *Behav Brain Res.* (1984): 11(2): 123–34.

Villablanca, J. R. "Counterpointing the Functional Role of the Forebrain and of the Brainstem in the Control of the Sleep-Waking System. *J Sleep Res.* (2004): 13(3): 179–208.

Zhu, M. Y., Vannier, J., Van Iten, H., and Zhao, Y. L. "Direct Evidence for Predation on Trilobites in the Cambrian." *Proc Biol Sci.* (2004): 271, Supplement 5: S277–80.

Zimmer, C. "Testing Darwin." *Discover* (2005): 26(2): 28–35.

Zimmer, C. *Evolution: The Triumph of an Idea.* New York: HarperCollins, 2001.

Stage 1: Sensorimotor

Stage 2: Preoperational

Stage 3: Concrete Operational

Stage 4: Formal Operational

—Jean Piaget's four stages of childhood development

CHAPTER V: Dreaming

Tracking the brain's developmental path through evolution has led us to a perspective on the influences and behaviors affecting brain development and the activities of its constituent parts. As we have learned, the brain is never more electrically active than when it is awake. This indicator of wakefulness in the brain, as we have also learned, is not exclusively caused by an animal's experiences in the physical world.

Diencephalon and Telencephalon

Waking experiences in the physical world cause distinct and measurable levels of electrical activity in the brain. During wakefulness, functional studies of the brain involving cognition experiments have shown elevated levels of glucose metabolism across several cortical regions. These signatures of a wakeful and thinking brain are the same signatures researchers have found in their extensive studies of the dreaming brain. The implication of all this is that the brain behaves and functions like a wakeful brain when it dreams. We know, from the last chapter, that dreaming is part of the diencephalon and telencephalon level of brain development. Therefore, the wakeful behavior and functions the brain engages when it dreams are those of the diencephalon and telencephalon.

Nothing in the study of the evolution of the human brain or the copious research on its structure suggests that dreaming alters the basic functions of the diencephalon and the telencephalon. Although a drop in our normal body temperature during sleep atonia appears to provide dream researchers evidence of altered function in the brainstem, this evidence has been misinterpreted. The appearance of lost homeostasis is caused by the function of the metencephalon and its suspension of somatosensory from the skin and musculature of the body during atonic sleep.

Sensory Disconnect

As we have explored in the previous chapter, the basic function of the diencephalon is to detect and respond effectively to affecting influences. This function is not changed by its arousal during atonic sleep. Although diencephalic function is immutable, its scope is not. During sleep atonia, the metencephalon separates the brain from its physical sources of sensory information. This severed connection limits the range of diencephalic function to nonphysical sources of sensory information. Other than sensory data detectable by sight or smell, the diencephalon does not receive sensory information from the physical environment. Without physical sensory input during atonic sleep, the wakeful diencephalon begins to process the residual effects of atonia on the structure of the brain, along with any detectable visual or olfactory data that has breached the electrochemical disturbance caused by the metencephalic release of muscle readiness. (See **Evolution: Muscle Readiness, Hypothalamus Psychology.**)

Visual and Olfactory Senses

Interestingly, if our eyelids open partially in a lit environment or our sinuses congest slightly during a dream, these sensations become part of the content of our dreams. One dream researcher, Dr. LaBerge, studied the effects of light on lucid dreaming and later marketed a device in the early 90s that used visual sensory perception to induce conscious lucidity during dreaming. In separate sleep studies, Dr. Carskadon and Dr. Badia linked physiological changes in heart rate and respiration during atonic sleep to the olfactory detection of peppermint. However, neither visual nor olfactory data is sufficient to cause physical wakefulness.

Tegmentum (Ascending Reticular Activating System)

The closing of our eyelids during atonic sleep stops most external imagery from entering our dreams. Our eyelids remain closed because they are not directly connected to the brain circuitry active during atonic sleep. Visual and olfactory information does not enter at the level of brain structure that stimulates wakefulness. Sounds and tactile stimulation can and do cause physical wakefulness during sleep atonia because they enter at the metencephalon level of brain structure. When aural and tactile receptors are sufficiently stimulated during atonia, a group of neurons in the tegmentum of the metencephalon—the ascending reticular activating system—initiate wakefulness by altering thalamic receptivity

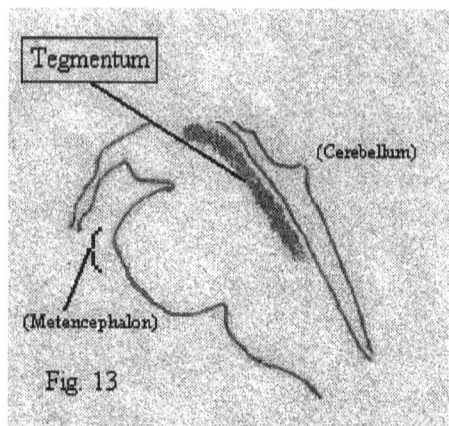

Fig. 13

to physical sensory data. The thalamus, as previously described, is the structure in the diencephalon through which all sensory data (except olfactory data) must initially pass before reaching the cortex. Although some sleep studies seem to contradict this, the neural activity of the tegmentum decreases and effectively isolates or disconnects the thalamus from sound and tactile sensory data during atonic sleep.

Tegmentum PET

Positron emission tomography (PET) studies of the tegmentum all show elevated activity during atonia, and EEG studies have produced theta waves and spontaneous electrical spikes suggestive of activity. However, PET studies do not account for the effect of atonic internalization of energy. This process arose as a survival strategy to preserve vital bodily systems through periods of extended privation during the metencephalic stage of brain evolution. The increased blood flow to the tegmentum seen in PET studies during atonia may merely reflect the preservation of the tegmentum, rather than its function.

Tegmentum EEG

Electroencephalograph (EEG) studies of the electrical activity of the tegmentum have produced results suggestive of its active function while the brain is dreaming. Researchers perceive the phasic electrical spikes between the tegmentum, the lateral geniculate, and the occipital lobe as evidence of ascending tegmentum function. In reality, the reverse is true. The electrical activity observed during atonia is an efferent echo from input to the nerves embedded in the metencephalon from superior brain structures. Although EEG studies suggest that the metencephalon is active through the tegmentum during atonic sleep, only the efferent nerve fibers embedded in its structure are truly active. (See **Evolution: Preparation Effect/REM.**)

Dreaming Process

During atonic sleep, dreaming arises in the cortex due to the effects of subcortical activity. We know this is how dreaming begins, because the cortex continuously registers slow-wave activity when its connections to its subcortical structure are severed. The likely source of the activity that initiates dreaming is the hypothalamus, through its afferent connections to the thalamus.

Active during atonic sleep, the hypothalamus regulates every vital system of the body and is responsive to influences impacting our drives, emotions, and survival. (See Chapter IV.) The thalamus instantly recognizes the influences it perceives during atonic arousal as nonphysical. Any influence that is not detected and encoded through the physical senses of the body is classified by the thalamus as nonphysical. (See Chapter III.)

The brain does not perceive nonphysical data arising from the hypothalamus as a physical need or a bodily threat. Therefore, this type of diencephalic stimulation does not arouse the wakeful responses of the body musculature governed by the metencephalon. When the metencephalic structures are intact and functioning normally, we do not physically act upon the nonphysical influences that resonate in our brainstems. However, this type of influence does arouse the assessment and response processes of the telencephalon.

Essence of Dreaming

Everything in the evolution and research of brain structure suggest that each succeeding structure of the central nervous system, from spinal cord to cortex, enhances the functions of preceding structure. The functions of the telencephalon enhance the functions of the diencephalon. This enhancement gives us the capacity to recall the past, anticipate the future, and devise behavioral responses in the present based on hindsight and foresight. This combination of hindsight and foresight is the very essence of dreaming. When thalamic perceptions of influences reach the cortex of the telencephalon during atonic sleep, they are given form, substance, and mental relevance.

Physical Laws and Logic

In an earlier chapter, we established dreams as information and said that in a sense, this information was meaningful. However, we made no distinction as to whether the meaningful information dreams seem to provide is useful information. When we examine the available evidence, we can distinctly determine that dreaming is a continuation of brain function during the vestigial arousal atonic sleep precipitates. In fulfilling its functional imperative, we now know that the dreaming brain is assessing and responding to nonphysical influences. This insight alone would be enough to establish dream information as useful, if not for the seeming incongruity of dreams with the laws and logic of physical experience and physical reality. Dreams do not conform to the rules of physical experience and reality for two basic reasons: dreams are not physical experiences and they do not occur in physical reality.

Nonphysical/Mental Influences

Empirically, dreams are mental manifestations of brain function during atonic sleep. The nonphysical influences affecting brain structure at the start of dreaming can only describe influences that exclusively impact brain function and the mind this function produces. In other words, it describes psychological rather than physiological influences. This is confirmed by their likely origin from hypothalamic sleep activity.

Consider the conundrum of trying to identify influences that do not have any physical attributes other than their effects on brain function. In your opinion, by what means is it reasonably possible for the brain to determine the nature of an influence it did not receive through its physical senses? The answer to this question also provides an answer to the question of whether dreams offer useful information.

Sensory Mapping

Solving the conundrum of identifying nonphysical influences is a primary function of the cortex. Physical experience alters cortical structure and can form neurological representations in the structure of the brain. New information about our experiences creates new neural connections. Much of the cortical structure behind the frontal lobe is devoted to this type of sensory mapping. Sensory mapping infers that the cortex identifies influences by the way those influences affect the structure of the brain. Although nonphysical influences may not have material substance, they do have effects. Our psychological sciences are dedicated to such effects. Essentially, the dreaming brain detects and identifies nonphysical influences—psychological influences—by the way those influences affect its structure.

Usefulness

We can now assert with some degree of certainty that our dreams may be useful indicators of the psychological effects of the influences affecting our wakeful brains during atonic sleep. However, we have yet to fully clarify how the brain selects the images it uses in dreams to identify the effects it detects. Clarification resides in how the brain uniformly collects and stores information about itself and its environment.

Material/Literal Distinction

All influences are distinguished by their physical nature and impact during physical wakefulness. This is a literal distinction. For example, we can distinguish a cigar by its appearance, smell, taste, and texture. These physical distinctions are delivered into the interpretive regions of the brain by the sensory connections between the brain and the eyes, nose, mouth, and other sensory receptors. To some of us, a cigar may be perceived as a symbol of wealth and power. However, symbolism is not a quality our physical senses encode. Symbolism is attached to our sensory experiences elsewhere in the brain. Therefore, to paraphrase Freud, a cigar is literally a cigar to our physical senses and to those regions of the brain that receive and interpret this physical information. Even influences that arise within the mind during physical wakefulness are perceived from a material, or literal, perspective.

Imagination/Literal Distinction

In our conscious minds, we can imagine all sorts of influences and experiences. However, what we imagine will always define something material and relevant to literal experience. Although, for example, we might envision a cigar sprouting wings and taking flight as a symbol of fleeting power, this would be a combination of literal images we mentally selected and linked to produce a vision of material significance. Uppermost in our conscious minds, a cigar with wings remains a cigar. In the conscious brain, all experience is interpreted from a literal perspective. This literal distinction of experience changes when we enter atonic sleep and our brains begin to dream.

Physical to Mental

The dreaming brain is a structure affected by nonphysical influences—influences of mental or psychological impact. To distinguish the nature of these influences, all the brain has at its disposal is its perception of their effects and a map of distinct physical effects it has amassed through life experience. When the brain detects effects of nonphysical impact during atonic sleep, it identifies those effects by overlaying them with its map of equivalent physical effects. Put more succinctly, the dreaming brain equates mental impact with physical impact. It defines the nature of a mental effect by substituting a physical effect of equal impact. For example, houses shelter our bodies and food satisfies their appetites. In the dreaming brain, houses may describe mental shelters and food the things that satisfy mental appetites. In our dreams, every image and every experience describes a distinct mental effect.

Mental Meaning

Every element of every dream we experience, regardless of our individuality, nationality, or ethnicity, describes something our brains perceive as a mental effect. The simplest way to understand our dream experiences is to prefix every element with the word "mental." For example, a dream about walking into a restaurant, having a seat, and eating some pie becomes a dream about mentally walking into a mental restaurant, having a mental seat, and mentally eating some mental pie. As an element in our dream, even presence describes a distinctly mental quality.

The Dreamer

The mental qualities we individually identify as components in our dream content are best described by the following passage from *The Dream Document: A Fundamental Guide to Dream Translation.*

> Consciousness is that mental quality in a living being that defines its existence. In humans, it is our sense of self and knowing that we exist. In our dreams, we are this abiding awareness of self that is cognizant of its distinction and existence apart from surrounding influence and experience. In your dreams, you are your consciousness. You are your all-encompassing awareness as a sentient being. As consciousness in your dreams, you represent that element of your being that travels between the gates of mental and physical reality.

As dreamers, we manifest the most essential element of dream content and human existence: consciousness.

Dreaming *vs.* Mental Peace

Tonic sleep is the most restful state of brain function, whereas atonic sleep arouses brain activity that disrupts this peaceful mental condition. In a sense, dreaming is an intrusion on the mental peace of tonic sleep. The images in our dreams describe our perceptions of what has intruded on our mental peace. The vestigial imperative of atonic wakefulness suggests that this intrusion on our peace affects our mental drives and sense of well-being. Early animals woke from proto-sleep either to feed themselves or to fend off predators. In the present day, this primal imperative during sleep has become its mental equivalent. Our dreams describe the influences that affect our mental appetite and well-being—influences that affect our mental peace. Consider the following dream:

My husband woke me up last week during the middle of the night and told me that he had dreamed that I told him I was leaving him to go off on a sea cruise with another man. It really upset him. Considering that we have been married for thirty-two years, it made me smile. Any ideas what the dream may have meant? By the way, he didn't see my new lover; I only told him that I was going off with another man.

The scenario of spousal infidelity is an obvious social threat of significant impact on the thirty-two-year marriage of the dreamer. It is likely that this dream describes influences impacting the well-being of the dreamer. However, to be certain of this perspective, we must translate this dream's imagery reliably.

Every dream translation should begin with unwavering certainty of the dreamer's role and of the general nature of dreams. Everything in a dream, including the dreamer, is how the brain assesses and responds to the mental effects it perceives when it arouses after tonic sleep. In the above dream, the dreamer is a mental assessment of himself. In his dream, he is his consciousness. Everything other than himself is how the dreamer's wakeful brain assessed the effects it detected upon arousal during atonic sleep.

Lasting *vs.* Transitory Effects

The effects of the influences we detect during sleep are the lingering psychological effects of life experience. We know this to be accurate, because life experience is our brain's only source of sensory information. Without this experience, our brains, like our muscles, atrophy through disuse. Life experience alters brain structure. The residual psychological effects we experience as dreams are akin to the behavioral effects that may be observed when the brain is surgically altered. Residual effects of our conscious experiences that manifest as dreams suggest that the overall focus of our dreams will most often involve influences of lasting, rather than transitory, effect. Influences that persist from conscious reality into dreams as images suggest the persistent, unresolved nature of those influences. This may explain why our dreams appear to involve some urgent issues from our life and not others. The issues absent from dream content suggest their transitory nature.

My husband woke me up last week during the middle of the night and told me he had dreamed that I...

As a manifestation of his consciousness, the dreamer perceives an affecting social influence characterized as his wife. In our dreams, people primarily signify the effects of our encounters with them. Socialization is a primary effect of our interactions with others. The dreamer's wife is likely one of his primary social influences. Her characterization in his dream suggests the impact of her influence on his consciousness. In his dream, she is not a literal depiction of her persona; she is his assessment of her impact on his mind. Her actions in the dream reflect the way the dreamer perceives he has been mentally impacted by her influence.

> *…I told him…*

The actions of the dreamer's wife do not describe something she literally said. Dreams are about mental effects; therefore, his wife's words describe the effect of something she might have expressed through other means, such as her behavior.

> *…I was leaving him to go off on a sea cruise with another man. It really upset him.*

In some way, the dreamer's wife has given him the impression that she has a social interest that will result in her abandonment of him, mentally or socially. The vocal introduction of "another man" in this dream is how the dreamer understands the compelling social influence leading his wife away from him.

> *By the way, he didn't see my new lover; I only told him that I was going off with another man.*

Whatever is unseen in a dream is not proven to the dreamer. The dreaming brain assesses and depicts only what it has clearly perceived. The visual, textural, and aural absence of another man suggests that the dreamer has not experienced any expression of a social intrusion on his marriage other than what he believes his wife has immaterially expressed. Consider the follow-up response of his wife to our translation of her husband's dream:

> *Yes, there could be some point in what you say. I have recently lost a lot of weight, and my husband keeps teasing me about other men finding me attractive. Perhaps this manifested itself in his dream. I am also going to be promoted into a high-profile position, so although he is pleased for me, he could be wondering how it will affect our personal lives. (He doesn't need to worry!)*

We now clearly understand that his wife's revived interest in her appearance gave the dreamer the impression that her behavior was not for his benefit. The dreamer was beginning to believe that his wife's social interests, unseen by him, would ultimately result in their social separation. Clearly, this dream describes the dreamer's perception of a threat to his social well-being. Any variation in our clarity on the general nature of dreams and dream characterizations would certainly have led us to a less precise translation than what we have here.

Characterization

Although our dreams are meaningful and useful forms of psychological information, they are only useful to the extent we are able to understand them and apply that understanding meaningfully to precise experiences in our life. By now, we should have a clear perspective on how the brain perceives the effects of influences during atonic sleep and how it identifies those effects through dream imagery. In the absence of physical sensory data during sleep atonia, our wakeful brains perceive and identify every influence by its effect on our mental nature. The brain identifies or characterizes each effect by comparing it to an equivalent physical effect it has previously mapped. In essence, dreams are mental effects characterized as physical experience. Our dreaming brains consistently characterize specific types of mental effects using specific types of dream imagery.

People

The people we encounter in our dreams consistently reflect the mental effects of social influence. Instead of representing themselves, dream-people reflect their impact on our mental nature. In the previous dream example, the dreamer's wife was how his dreaming brain perceived and characterized the lingering effect of a social encounter with her. However, the people in our dreams are frequently not evidence of our direct social encounters with them in our conscious life. Consider the following dream:

> *I had this dream that I was with my best friend from high school and we were lined up at a counter to order our lunch. It was a cafeteria-type restaurant. I don't recognize it in the dream. I was going to order bacon and eggs. This is my favorite breakfast in real life. Then my grandmother appeared beside me in the line. She had her pink housecoat on. In real life, she has passed away. I remember that my pants fell down and I was naked. I felt so embarrassed. I was trying to fix them, but it was so difficult in the dream. Finally, I did succeed at getting my pants on. Then my grandmother had an*

*asthma attack and I was going frantically through her purse and
found the puffer. When she took it, we both felt relief.*

The dreamer's best friend from high school and her grandmother were people
who were not in the dreamer's life at the time of the dream. Her best friend was a
person with whom she had lost contact for several years, and her grandmother
was deceased. Their absence from her conscious life suggests that their presence in
her dream was likely not a result of the dreamer's ongoing conscious relationship
with them. Several dream authorities perceive this type of imagery as indicative of
some aspect of the dreamer's psyche. Particularly, advocates of Jung's analysis
methods perceive the people, places, and things in our dreams as representations
of ourselves. According to this method, the dreamer's best friend and grandmother are creations of the dreamer's mind and probably aspects of the dreamer
herself. However, this perception of her dream imagery is not precise.

The evidence clearly indicates that dreams are not mental creations; they are
perceptions of the residual mental effects of the influences persisting from conscious life into atonic sleep. Dreams are how the brain perceives and identifies the
resonant mental effects of conscious life experience that sleep has not abated.
Dream imagery involving familiar people identifies the persistent effects of social
influences familiar to the dreamer. Imagery involving people absent from the life
of the dreamer also identifies the effects of familiar social influences. They identify the way certain social influences in life trigger the familiar mental effects of
other influences.

Dreams are how the brain perceives the effects of influences during sleep.
Although the trigger for an effect can be any latent influence from a dreamer's
sphere of conscious experience, the effects themselves are specific. Therefore, any
attempt to translate a dream is an attempt to identify specific mental effects.
Specifically, people identify the mental effects triggered by social influences. They
are how our dreaming brains perceive the lingering mental impact of our conscious interaction or relationship with others. In the dream example provided, the
dreamer's best friend and grandmother identify the way her mind has been specifically affected by some aspect of her social experiences.

*...I was with my best friend from high school and we were lined up
at a counter to order our lunch.*

This portion of the dream suggests that some social experience has had a mental
affect upon the dreamer that was like being in line with her best friend from high
school, waiting to order lunch.

> *Then my grandmother appeared beside me in the line. She had her*
> *pink housecoat on.*

Again, some social experience resonant with the sudden appearance of her grand-mother in a pink housecoat has had an impact on the dreamer's mind.

Although the details of the dreamer's conscious relationship with her best friend from high school and her grandmother might provide a clearer picture of the particular mental effects they identify in her dream, those effects can be sur-mised from what we already know. For example, we know that a primary mental impact of having friends is a sense of social acceptance. When a friend becomes a best friend, this adds an extra degree of intimacy and trust to the impact of social acceptance. Therefore, best-friend imagery describes the mental impact of inti-mate or personal social acceptance. In the dream above, this imagery describes some sense of personal social acceptance the dreamer has experienced.

Assessing the mental impact of having a grandmother can be similarly facili-tated through a general perception of grandparents as older and more experienced than parents. Generally, an impact of age and experience is wisdom. In the above example, the sudden appearance of the dreamer's grandmother might identify the emergence of social wisdom (age and experience) in the mind of the dreamer. This suggests that some social experience has aroused a sense of social wisdom in the mind of the dreamer. Whether this or any other translation of human imagery is precise depends on the mental influences suggested by every other dream detail.

The relevance of dreams to the experiences and influences of conscious life is not borne solely by the people in them; it is conveyed by every aspect of dream content. Every dream characterization—everything the dreamer sees, hears, taste, smells, feels, thinks, and does in dreams—identifies some mental effect. The more mental effects we decode from dream content, the more we are able to determine what relevance a dream may have to a dreamer's conscious experience.

Places

If the dreamer's persona reflects the element of consciousness in a dream, the dreamer's location in a dream describes the effects enveloping that consciousness. Each time a place is referenced in a dream, it describes how the dreamer perceives some enveloping mental experience. For example, "my best friend from high school" describes the sense of personal social acceptance the dreamer has acquired through the effects of an enveloping mental experience identified by high school.

The enveloping mental effects suggested by the places mentioned, seen, or entered in dream content are described by the general nature of physical experience in those places. In physical reality, high school is a structured environment of educational and social experiences. In dream content, high school identifies the enveloping mental effects of social learning experiences. Here, "education" has become "learning" in the context of the dream, because learning is ultimately the mental impact of education. Therefore, "my best friend from high school" describes the sense of personal social acceptance the dreamer has acquired from what she has learned through her experiences.

Another place referenced in our dream example was a cafeteria-type restaurant. As with all imagery, when the dreamer provides no additionally descriptive information, we begin our translation of this imagery with what we generally know about the type of place depicted. Cafeterias and restaurants are generally places where people go to experience meals or satisfy their appetites. The mental impact of eating food is the experience of an inwardly satisfying effect. In our dream example, being in a cafeteria-type restaurant probably describes the ambient mental effect of experiences in which the dreamer has engaged to satisfy something she inwardly desires. Generally, structures or places a dreamer sees or enters describe the ambient effects of enveloping experiences. Structures, specifically, identify the ambient effects of structured social experiences and environments. The nature of those experiences and environments suggested by dream content is identified by the type of structure depicted; *e.g.*, a high school suggest an environment of learning experiences, and a restaurant symbolizes an environment of inwardly satisfying experiences.

Things

The nature of dream content is limited only by the mind of the dreamer. Whatever a dreamer envisions and experiences on a conscious level can also arise as dream content. This shows the limitless nature of dream content and the improbability of any book ever containing definitive translations for every conceivable dream characterization. Although numerous, the complexities and nuances of life experience manifesting as dream imagery are discernable through the relativity of mental effect to physical experience.

...we were lined up at a counter to order our lunch.

Like everything else in a dream, the actions of the dreamer describe some mental effect. The effect of waiting in a line is generally the anticipation of what awaits at its end. In her dream, the dreamer was in line to order lunch. In physical reality, lunch is usually an interval of nourishment amid an experience of purposeful endeavor. The mental impact of lunch is the satisfaction of a inner yearning amid a respite from a purposeful experience. In combination, "we were lined up at a counter to order our lunch" simply describes the dreamer's anticipation of satisfying some yearning she has, during a respite from some purposeful pursuit.

> *I was going to order bacon and eggs. This is my favorite breakfast in real life.*

In her dream, the dreamer yearns for her favorite breakfast, bacon and eggs. Although each food selection describes a separate and distinct mental effect, her overall description of them as "breakfast" suggests that her inner yearning has come after a period of self-denial. We derive this translation from the nature of fasting suggested by the description of breaking a fast.

> *Then my grandmother appeared...She had her pink housecoat on...I remember that my pants fell down and I was naked. I felt so embarrassed. I was trying to fix them, but it was so difficult in the dream. Finally, I did succeed at getting my pants on.*

We generally select the things we wear in conscious life for either adornment or utility. Clothes enhance your self-image, protect your modesty, and shield your body from adverse climate conditions. The comparable mental effects suggested by clothing perceived in dream content are either the projection or protection of self-image or social image. The pink housecoat worn by the dreamer's grandmother projects something distinct about the sense of social wisdom emerging in the mind of the dreamer. However, the dreamer's problem with her pants suggests something distinct about the dreamer's self-image. The mental impact of anything that falls suggests a failure of those things to maintain the position from which they fell. The general impact of nakedness is the perception of being intimately exposed and vulnerable. Thus, "my pants fell down and I was naked" describes the sense of vulnerability and exposure the dreamer has experienced through a failure to maintain some aspect of her self-image.

> *Then my grandmother had an asthma attack and I was going frantically through her purse and found the puffer. When she took it, we both felt relief.*

The actions of the dreamer in her dream describe her mental efforts. In the above dream segment, her mental efforts are focused on finding a remedy for a threatening affliction affecting the social wisdom suggested by the imagery of her grandmother. Generally, asthma suggest a threat to life because it obstructs the respiratory function of the body. In the context of a dream, an endangerment to life is an endangerment to vitality. The grandmother's asthma attack identifies a threat to the vitality of the dreamer's social wisdom.

Translating the individual people, places, and things in a dream is informative, but not as useful to our understanding of a dream's overall relevance to the life of a dreamer. The overall relevance of a dream resides in piecing together the individual effects suggested by its imagery in the order described by the dreamer. Consider the following overall translation originally rendered to the dreamer, and her response:

Translation:

In your dream, your best friend could describe the friend you are to yourself, or the sort of friendships you enjoy most. The cafeteria describes the social experiences enveloping your thoughts as represented within the dream. The cafeteria may represent the experiences in your life that you have engaged to satisfy your inner yearnings. Your yearning for breakfast food in the dream describes a deeply felt desire that may have surfaced after a lengthy period of self-denial. It describes your desire for an inwardly satisfying experience after having endured a period of unfavorable social circumstances.

Your grandmother's presence describes the influence of traditional wisdom and experience. She may represent the way your thoughts are influenced by the social ideas and mores you were taught as a child. It is interesting that your grandmother appears as your pants fall. This could suggest how the ideas your grandmother reflects influence your self-image. In some way, you may have failed to maintain a social image or sense of self that is beyond reproach. Being naked below the waist could describe your sense of how you have become vulnerable or immodest. Your effort to cover up could describe an effort to not be perceived as intimately vulnerable, exposed, or immodest. Your grandmother's seizure and your effort to supply her need may describe your efforts to sustain or resuscitate the social ideas she personifies.

Response:

I agree with what you said. You are totally right when you say my yearning for breakfast food describes a deeply felt desire after a period of self-denial. I have been through some bad experiences. I have isolated myself to reflect. My situation has made me totally vulnerable, and I feel exposed. I feel it's for my own well-being to cover it up. I think that if anyone had to go through the experiences that I had to face, they would be trying to cover it up also. I agree with what you said about my grandmother. This is very true.

Although the dreamer provided few details to substantiate the translation she received, her positive response suggests that the translated effects of her dream may have had some resonance with her conscious experience. However, the validity of a dream's translation should not be dependent on a dreamer's responses or upon any intimate knowledge of the dreamer's life. The validity and reliability of dream translation relies on a comprehensive knowledge of the neurological nature of dreaming and dream characterization.

*   *   *

Neurologically, dreaming is how the brain responds to the resonant effects of conscious life experience that persist in the structure of the brain during atonic sleep. This description of dreaming (and the evidence in evolution and brain research we have examined in previous chapters) supports a new paradigm for our understanding of the brain and the mind it produces. In the next chapter, we will examine this new model of brain function and mental structure suggested by dreaming and its supporting research.

REFERENCE

Badia, P., Wesensten, N., Lammers, W., Culpepper, J., and Harsh, J. "Responsiveness to Olfactory Stimuli Presented in Sleep." *Physiol Behav.* (1990): 48(1): 87–90.

Carskadon, M. A. and Herz, R. S. "Minimal Olfactory Perception during Sleep: Why Odor Alarms Will Not Work for Humans." *Sleep* (2004): 27(3): 402–5.

Crochet, S. and Sakai, K. "Effects of Microdialysis Application of Monoamines on the EEG and Behavioural States in the Cat Mesopontine Tegmentum." *Eur J Neurosci.* (1999): 11(10): 37–38.

Horgan, J. "Lucid Dreaming Revisited." *Omni* (1994): 16(12): 44–46.

Howell, K. D. *The Dream Document: A Fundamental Guide to Dream Translation.* Lincoln: Authors Choice Press, 2001.

Kolb, B. and Whishaw, I. Q. *Fundamentals of Human Neuropsychology* (4th ed.). New York: Worth, 2000.

Maloney, K. J., Mainville, L., and Jones, B. E. "Differential c-Fos Expression in Cholinergic, Monoaminergic, and GABAergic Cell Groups of the Pontomesencephalic Tegmentum after Paradoxical Sleep Deprivation and Recovery." *J Neurosci.* (1999): 19(8): 3057–3072.

Maquet, P. "Functional Neuroimaging of Normal Human Sleep by Positron Emission Tomography." *J. Sleep Res.* (2001): 9: 207–231.

Mazzilotta, J. C., Phelps, M. E., Miller, J., and Kuhl, D.E. "Tomographic Mapping of Human Cerebral Metabolism: Normal Unstimulated State." *Neurology* (1981): 31(5): 503–16.

Perry, B. D. "Childhood Experiences and the Expression of Genetic Potential: What Childhood Neglect Tells Us about Nature and Nurture." *Brain and Mind* (2002): 3: 79–100.

Portas, C. M., *et al.* "Auditory Processing across the Sleep-Wake Cycle: Simultaneous EEG and fMRI Monitoring in Humans." *Neuron.* (2000): 28: 991–999.

Shouse, M. N. and Siegel, J. M. "Pontine Regulation of REM Sleep Components in Cats: Integrity of the Pedunculopontine Tegmentum (PPT) Is Important for Phasic Events but Unnecessary for Atonia during REM Sleep." *Brain Res.* (1992): 571: 50–63.

Tootell, R. B. H., *et al.* "Functional Anatomy of Macaque Striate Cortex II: Retinotopic Organization." *J. Neurosci.* (1988): 8: 1531.

Simple truths are a relief from grand speculations.

—Vauvenargues

CHAPTER VI: Function and Structure

Several chapters ago, we began our investigation of dreaming with a simple truth:

> Psychology, as it relates to the processes and products of mental activity, is empirically impossible without an underlying neurological structure as its progenitor…dreams, as probable psychological products, are not possible without the neurological structure we have evolved to support dreaming.

In later chapters, we established the psychological basis of dreams through their origin in brain structures whose functions reveal another truth:

> Nothing happens in the brain that is not a product of some neurological influence.

Through this truth, we determined brain activity to be an effect of neurological influences both internal and external to the sensory systems of the body. This was particularly important to our understanding of dreaming, because it distinguished dreams as products of influences rather than as byproducts of spontaneous neurological activity. Specifically, we found that dreaming is a consequence of activity in the brainstem arising from the biological and functional imperatives of its constituent structures. When we examined the primary imperative of these constituent structures, we uncovered a more cogent perspective of brain function and mental structure than the amalgam of perspectives rendered in the last century.

Functional and Structural Review

When we examine the path of the human brain through evolution, we find evidence at every succeeding level of brain structure that its development was induced by the acquisition of new sensory systems. The evidence suggests that the brain evolved as it became more perceptive. We begin this functional review of the brain and its mental constructs with another truth, established in earlier chapters:

> Everything in the evolution and research of brain structure suggests that each succeeding structure of the central nervous system, from spinal cord to cortex, enhances the functions of preceding structures.

Myelencephalon

For the reasons cited above, the sense of touch introduction, followed by taste, at the myelencephalon (Fig. 14) level of brain structure was pivotal to human brain evolution. Touch and taste afferents at this level of brain development in contemporary animals provide reliable evidence of the earliest point in prehistory when early animals began to make clear distinctions about their sensory environments and the nutrients they derived from those environments. The sense of touch suggests that they became responsive to their environments, and the sense of taste suggests that they became selective in their responses.

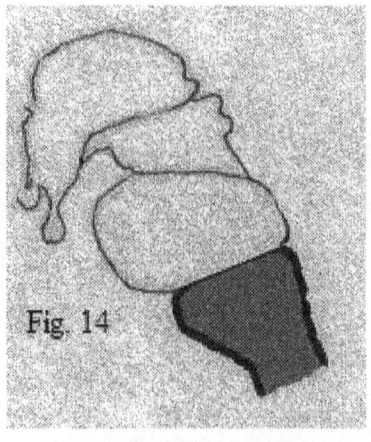

Fig. 14

The new behaviors these sensory perceptions influenced increased the energy requirements of early animals, and subsequently their requirements for nutrients.

During periods of privation, early animals developed survival behaviors to conserve their energy reserves until resources became available. The metencephalon and the sleep process prevalent in present-day animals originated from those behaviors.

Metencephalon

The process of dreaming begins during sleep with a partial isolation of the brain from the sensory systems of the body by neuronal structures in the metencephalon (Fig. 4). All tactile, taste, and aural data must pass through this segment of brainstem to reach the upper regions of the central nervous system. The metencephalon separates the brain from the sensory information that traverses its structure during the atonic sleep processes it regulates. Visual and olfactory sensory data does not enter the brain through the metencephalon, and therefore remain unaffected by metencephalic sleep functions. The isolation of the brain from its palpable sources of sensory information during atonic sleep brings us to another cogent perspective of overall brain function and mental structure:

> The unconscious mind, as dreaming shows, is a product of brain function in isolation from metencephalic contact (touch, taste, and sound) with physical reality.

This perspective is a variation on the nature of the mind described in earlier chapters as a product of brain function. Here, the unconscious mind is a product of brain function in isolation from contact with physical reality. The metencephalon establishes the brain's physical connection to reality by supplying the energy that afferent neural pathways require to deliver physical sensory information to the brain. This delivery of sensory data is periodically suspended when the metencephalon engages its atonic sleep processes.

Tonic Sleep (Muscle Readiness)

During sleep, the metencephalon mediates tonic and atonic activity in the musculature of the body; it regulates muscle readiness. Sleep begins with our musculature in a ready, tonic state. This muscle tonicity is a remnant of our primal past. It is associated with the readiness and vigilance early animals required in order to arouse quickly from a state of inactivity to engage in survival behavior. During the dreaming phase of sleep, the metencephalon releases the body's musculature from this condition. This released, or atonic, state of muscle readiness is another behavioral remnant of our primal past.

Atonic Sleep (Energy Management)

Sleep primarily evolved as a function of the metencephalon to conserve energy during limited periods of physical inactivity and food privation. The evidence suggests that the metencephalic release of muscle tone (atonia) during sleep was adopted by early animals as a strategy to sustain life during extended periods of inactivity and privation. This was accomplished by channeling energy away from the musculature and into organs more vital to survival. This metencephalic system of energy management was subsequently enhanced by the development of the hypothalamus.

Intermediary Brainstem (Mesencephalon)

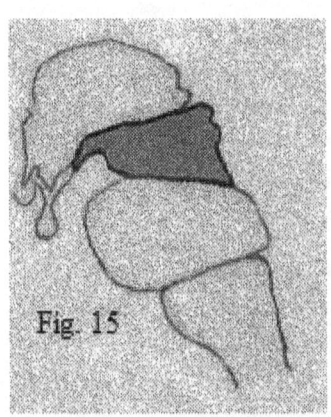

Fig. 15

The hypothalamus is the most primitive constituent structure of the diencephalic (Fig. 5) segment of brainstem. In the brainstem, the diencephalon is contiguous with the metencephalon through the mesencephalon (Fig. 15). The mesencephalon is the uppermost portion of the metencephalon, extending into the diencephalon. This extension compensates for the displacement of the superior colliculi (Fig. 16) from the diencephalic to the mesencephalic brainstem segment. The superior colliculi is a bilateral diencephalic substructure that receives visual information from the optic tract via the lateral geniculate body. Essentially, the mesencephalon is an intermediary segment of brainstem comprising both metencephalic and diencephalic structures.

Sound/Locomotion/Cerebellum

The evidence suggests that as early animals became more perceptive, they developed new behaviors and evolved brain structures to mediate those behaviors efficiently. The entry of aural sensory data at the metencephalic level of brain structure (in contemporary animals) provides evidence that early animals began to locomote at the metencephalic stage in brain evolution. The perception of sound indicates locomotion in these animals at this stage because its introduction suggests a survival advantage that probably required orienting toward and away from sources of sound. This behavior is supported at the metencephalic level by the cerebellum (Fig. 9) and its extensively researched association with balanced locomotion. (See Chapter IV, Tactile Sense and Aural Sense)

Hypothalamus (Energy Management Enhancement)

The energy demands of locomotion increase as animals engage in more complex movements and behaviors. The hypothalamus (Fig. 6) evolved in the structure of the brain after the appearance of hearing, when animals began to engage these movements and behaviors. This infers the intimate involvement of hypothalamic development with the energy management required by the new and increasing behaviors early animals were adapting. The complexity of these behaviors and their energy demands is reflected by the drives and physical processes the hypothalamus mediates in contemporary animals. (See Chapter IV, Hypothalamus.)

In contemporary animals, including humans, the metencephalon's cessation of muscle tone during sleep causes elevated neural activity and energy uptake in the brain, from the hypothalamus to the cortex. This effect of metencephalic energy management essentially results in the arousal of brain function during sleep. Through this arousal, we have reached yet another simple truth:

> Nothing in the study of the evolution of the human brain or in the copious research on its structure suggests that dreaming alters the basic functions of the diencephalon and the telencephalon.

Dreaming is the arousal of neural activity in the brain during atonic sleep. All research evidence indicates wakeful activity in the structures above the metencephalon during atonia. Although the metencephalon's cyclical cessations isolate the brain from wakeful contact with physical reality during sleep, the functional imperatives of the brain's remaining structures are not changed by this process when they become active during atonia. Although atonic sleep isolates the hypothalamus from the musculature of the body, the energy control its functions enhance remains intact in all the other systems of the body it has evolved to mediate.

Psychology

The evidence shows that the hypothalamus evolved as an enhancement to energy management when early animals became more mobile and engaged in increasingly sophisticated behaviors. This behavioral sophistication, as evidenced by the drive-related functions of the hypothalamus in contemporary animals, denotes the emergence of a psychology in early species at the hypothalamic level of brain evolution. For example, the sexual drive mediated by the hypothalamus in contemporary species suggests the hypothalamic emergence, in ancestral species, of socially connective behaviors to procure and maintain reproductive associations. Socially connective behaviors are reliable indicators of an adaptive psychology. The arousal of the hypothalamus at the beginning of sleep atonia essentially shows the psychological basis of dreaming in brain functions. (See Chapter IV, Hypothalamus Sexuality)

Superior Colliculi (Sight)

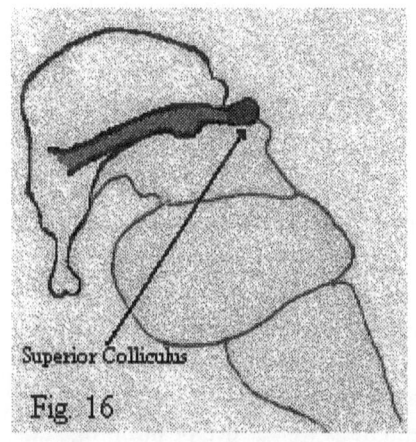

Superior Colliculus

Fig 16

Facilitated by efficient energy management, increased mobility extended the sensory experiences of early animals. This led to the acquisition of sight perception and the behavioral advances and brain structures the visual sense arouses. The coordination of facial afferents (cranial nerve V) with oculomotor efferents (cranial nerves III, IV, and VI) through the metencephalon in contemporary animals suggests that sight acquisition through the diencephalon (cranial nerve II) developed as an enhancement to tactile sensory perception.

The enhancement of sight arrived in primitive brain structure, after the hypothalamus, through the visual pathways leading to the superior colliculi. Although understated in previous chapters, sight perception is responsible for all growth of brain structure subsequent to the hypothalamus. Sight perception gave early animals the ability to engage in behaviors independent of instinct. Instead of merely reacting to taste, touch, and sound, they were able to act proactively through visual confirmation. Visual sensory input gave primal animals the ability to coordinate behavioral choices based on what they saw rather than what they tasted, felt, or heard. This behavioral adaptation spurred the development of the first formal brain.

Thalamus (Proto-brain)

The thalamus (Fig. 7), with its left/right hemisphere and interthalamic adhesion (Fig. 8) characteristics of the modern brain, was the first structure to assume the function of a proper brain. In early animals, as in contemporary species, this proto-brain was and remains the collection center for nearly all sensory data entering the brain. All incoming sensory information (except olfactory data) must first pass through the thalamus before entering the cerebrum. Although olfactory data enters parts of the telencephalon directly via the paleocortex, the thalamus subsequently receives olfactory afferents via its dorsomedial nucleus and other brain structures, including the hippocampus, the amygdala, and the hypothalamus. In early species, the thalamus would have enhanced behavior by coordinating taste, tactile, and sound data with visual data to arrive at behavioral choices advantageous to survival. For example, these animals might have conserved energy by limiting their instinctive reactions to those sensory affecting influences they could visually identify as having some survival impact.

Basal Ganglia

As behavioral choices became more coordinated through sight, movement gained more precision. The indiscriminant limb movement associated with sightless behavior was subdued by the development of the basal ganglia (Fig. 10) in the telencephalon. (See Chapter IV: Telencephalon.) Together with sight, the basal ganglia enhanced the precision of the behavioral responses early animals coordinated through the thalamus. In contemporary species, this structure permits smooth and steady arm, leg, and head movement as well as eye positioning. The basal ganglia facilitate our ability to smoothly and precisely orient and target our limb movements.

Amygdala

When animals acquired the capacity to coordinate physical sensory information visually, their ability to distinguish influences of survival impact became more efficient. This distinction of survival-affecting influences arose in the brain through the amygdala (Fig. 11b). The amygdala is the first structure of the limbic system (Fig. 11a) in the telencephalon region of the mammalian brain. In modern mammals, this structure has been shown to promote learning and long-term emotional memory. In early animals, the amygdala enhanced their recognition of survival-affecting influences by associating the sensory markers of those influences with previously sustained emotional effects. Associating survival influences in this manner enhanced the ability of these animals to coordinate sensory information and make secure behavioral choices based on the emotional effects persisting from prior experience.

Olfactory Bulb

Millions of years before the acquisition of sight, animals maintained contact with their ambient environments through taste perception. Sustaining such contact grew ever more important to their survival as they became increasingly proactive and their experiences widened through sight perception. Feeding and maintaining ambient sensory perception through the same orifice became an impractical survival design in their widening and increasingly predaceous environments. As a result, these animals evolved a separate orifice for the detection of the ambient sensory data occluded by feeding. In modern animals, the nasal passages and the olfactory bulb (Fig. 11a) reflect the orifices and subsequent brain structure early animals evolved to maintain ambient contact with their sensory environments.

Hippocampus

The olfactory bulb is the second most important structure of the limbic system. Its development enhanced sensory and behavioral coordination, which sight initiated, by adding the perception of scent to the widening experiences of early animals. After acquiring scent perception, these animals gained the capacity to recognize influences in their environments by scent, based on prior experience. This recognition resulted in the development of the hippocampus (Fig. 11a). The hippocampus, which is the final structure of the limbic system in this review, promotes learning and long-term memory in contemporary animals. It has been shown to promote spatial memory in scent-dependent animals. In early animals, this structure's connection to the olfactory bulb helped them to mentally retain the survival significance of scent-related effects.

Memory

From the moment animals began to experience emotional and olfactory effects, they began to develop brain structures to sustain the mental significance of those effects to their survival. First they developed an amygdala to mentally sustain the survival significance of the emotions attached to their experiences; then they developed a hippocampus to sustain the mental impact of their olfactory experiences. The mental significance these structures caused to persist in the minds of early animals enhanced their ability to make secure behavioral choices by promoting retrospection based on the resonant mental affects of prior experience. When a link between these structures formed to complete the limbic system, their functions combined to create the rudiments of memory. Because of memory, early animals became familiar with their habitats and were able to extend their cycle of wakefulness after proto-sleep into dream sleep.

Cortex

As the succession of prior brain developments establishes, the cortex (Fig. 12) arose as an enhancement to the functions of the brain structures preceding its development. The capacity to coordinate sensory information with behavioral choices, tempered by the mental effects sustained through prior experience, led to an expansion in brain development unlike any before. The resulting cortical structures enhanced the brain's ability to mediate sensory and behavioral experiences by extending the brain's capacity to sort, assess, coordinate, and store sensory and behavioral information. This is accomplished in the cortex by its capacity to map, within its structure, all sensory and sensorimotor experience.

Sensory Experience

The debate over the causes of human brain development is now at its end. Brain evolution, as the evidence plainly provides, followed a path laid by sensory acquisition. Beginning with touch, sensory perception enhanced the experiences of early animals and caused brain growths leading to behaviors more adaptive to their survival. The effect of sensory deprivation on brain growth and function in modern animals proves the significance of sensory experience to cortical development. Domesticated animals, for example, experience as much as a thirty-five percent reduction of growth in their visual cortexes (occipital lobes), compared to non-domesticated animals. Presumably, the visual experiences of domesticated animals are not as rich or varied as those of wild animals.

Divergent Brains

The path of sensory acquisition that the human brain marched to its current stage of development is not the path traveled by the brains of other animals. Nevertheless, sensory perception influenced brain development in all animals. In other animals, brain evolution was dictated by how their ancestral species exploited the survival advantages of the sensory systems their primitive brains acquired. For example, the olfactory epithelium in canines contains an estimated eighteen receptors per square centimeter, compared to four in humans. This suggests that canine ancestors, at some point in prehistory, began to exploit the survival advantages of scent more effectively than did human ancestors. Consequently, contemporary canines have a relatively larger area of brain architecture devoted to sensing scent.

Sensory perception enhanced brain development and continues to affect brain anatomy. Touch, taste, sound, sight, and smell are how the brain determines the nature of its reality. How the brain perceives reality is determined by the way sensory information enters it structure.

Physical Reality

Physical reality is distinguished by the physical sensory information arriving in the brain through the metencephalon. Physical sensory data arrives as tactile and sound perceptions directly from the metencephalon and indirectly as taste and additional tactile perceptions from the myelencephalon, through the metencephalon. The sensory influences introduced into the brain through these structures are encoded by afferent connections from the physical sensory arrays of the body, excluding those involving sight and smell.

All sensory experiences and brain activity occurring during the active state of metencephalic function are perceived by the brain as occurrences in physical reality. Although sight and scent are not encoded by the afferent pathways through the metencephalon, this data is also perceived as physical experience when the metencephalon is active. This perception of visual and olfactory data as physical experience during metencephalic arousal is an effect of thalamic function. The thalamus produces this effect by coordinating this data with the tactile, taste, and sound data it receives through the metencephalon. Visual and olfactory data that is experienced during metencephalic dormancy becomes part of dream content and is not perceived as a product of physical experience.

Mental Experience

Mental experience is the awareness within the brain produced by brain function. Thought, imagination, and dreaming are all mental experiences. However, these experiences are not all the same. The brain integrates mental experience with physical reality when the metencephalon is active. The hallmarks of physical experience, which metencephalic function brings into the brain, are interspersed with the mental activity comprising our thoughts and imagination when we are conscious. This association of thought and imagination with physical experience explains why these mental experiences are easier to recall than dreams.

Long-term Memory

All experience is processed in short-term memory. Experiences that occur when the brain is connected to physical reality eventually become part of long-term memory. The long-term memory of experiences with physical impact gave early animals a survival advantage. Consequently, the brain processes and stores physical experience for the long term. When thought and imagination are mingled with the experience of physical reality through an active metencephalon, they are processed and stored in long-term memory with their physical accompaniment. Our thoughts and imagined experiences, occurring as they do when we are consciously awake, are easier to remember because they are accompanied by physical experience. However, dreams are not as easy to remember, because they are not accompanied by true physical experience, as we are not connected to physical reality by an active metencephalon.

Short-term Memory

Most scientists agree that short-term memory experiences are intended to be just that—short-term. They believe that some products of brain function were never meant to be sustained long. However, the evolution of memory suggests that this belief is not entirely precise.

Memory evolved as the brains of early animals gained the ability to sustain the survival significance of the mental influences associated with their physical experiences. Through the amygdala and hippocampus, these animals were able to retain the mental effects caused by experiences of material consequence to their survival. Mental experiences of no material consequence had no impact on ancestral survival; therefore, nonphysical experiences of no material impact escape the mental retention of contemporary animals.

Prefrontal Cortex

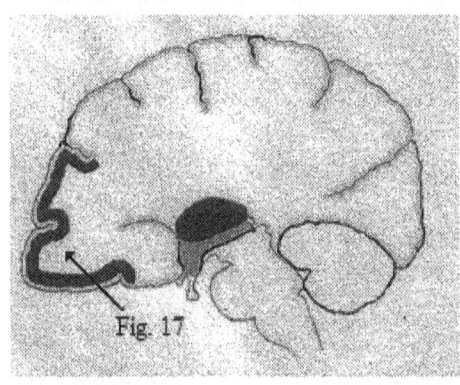

Fig. 17

In the human brain, the assessment of consequences is a primary function of the prefrontal cortex (Fig. 17). Whenever the prefrontal cortex is damaged, sufferers display a lack of interest in consequences or an inability to assess the consequences of their actions. This profoundly significant prefrontal ability is poorly understood by current science. For example, extensive functional studies of the prefrontal cortex in schizophrenic patients show diminished or depressed activity of a kind found when a normal brain experiences dreaming. This has led researchers to associate the supposed delusional nature of schizophrenia and dreaming with prefrontal dysfunction, when in reality it is not suggestive of a functional disorder in this area of the brain.

Ancestrally, only influences of material or physical consequence reached the prefrontal cortex and permanent memory processing. Prefrontal activity is depressed during dreaming because physical experience does not enter the brain as it does when the metencephalon is active. An active metencephalon causes the merger of physical experience with mental experience. This does not occur during sleep atonia. The prefrontal cortex is primed to respond only to input accompanying physical experience, because ancestrally, physical experience was the only experience of consequence to survival. Dreaming does not involve physical experience; therefore, dreaming does not arouse the prefrontal cortex. This suggests that the depressed prefrontal activity in the cortices of schizophrenics and the dreamlike imagery these patients experience are likely caused by an occlusion in the flow of physical sensory data from the metencephalon through the brainstem—an occlusion similar to what occurs when the brain is dreaming.

Dreaming

Dreaming is caused by arousal in the brain, beginning with the hypothalamus through the dormancy of metencephalic function. Because dreaming begins with hypothalamic arousal, dreams primarily reflect the mental effects of drive and survival-related influences. When its heightened energy regulatory functions are engaged during atonia, the hypothalamus causes an ascending cascade of mental effects from its structure in the diencephalon to those of the telencephalon. When these effects reach the telencephalon, the cortex engages its mapping functions to sort, assess, coordinate, and store the sensory information carried by the effects it detects. Although this process produces the sensations and sensory perceptions of physical experience, it is not recognized as such by the cortex. Without the afferent markers of physical sensory data from the metencephalon, the cortex processes these hypothalamus-inspired mental effects exclusively as mental experience. As purely mental experiences, dreams do not arouse the frontal cortex and are not processed and stored as permanent memory. This explains why the recollection of some dream details escapes long-term memory when we wake in physical reality.

Generally, we do not remember our dream experiences in detail or for very long because they do not contain the markers of physical experience. However, our brain's efforts to coordinate its mental experiences with its awakening metencephalic function, upon physical arousal, moves some of our dream experiences into long-term memory. When we remember our dreams in detail, it is a testament to the speed at which our brain is able to map its mental experiences with the physical perceptions aroused through our waking metencephalic function.

Dreaming vs. Conscious Experience

The distinction in brain function between the initiate of dreaming and that of conscious experience has profound implications. Conscious brain activity initiates through metencephalic arousal while dreaming involves hypothalamic stimulation. Of the two, the metencephalon is the most primitive. This suggests that the influences upon dream content arise from a brain structure more recent in our evolution than the structure that mediates our connection to conscious experience. The implication of this is profound in that our dreaming brain is influenced by a structure of more advanced function than our conscious brain. This influence supports a perspective of dreaming as a more advanced state of brain function than physical consciousness.

Dream Characterization

The brain characterizes dream content by equating mental experience with physical experience. This occurs as the metencephalon arouses from dormancy and the brain becomes consciously active. When the metencephalon arouses, the thalamus attempts to reconcile the brain's mental experiences with the physical perceptions arriving in the thalamus from the metencephalon. The mental effects atonia initiates produce mental experience, and the thalamus coordinates all experiences; therefore, reconciliation of mental experience with physical experience remains a function of the thalamus.

Dream Recall

The experience of dreaming is dissimilar to the mental process involving dream recall. When the brain is dreaming, it is isolated from physical sensory input. The effects that become dreams or mental experience in the cortex originate from the hypothalamus via the thalamus during atonic sleep. After forwarding them to the cortex, the thalamus re-experiences these hypothalamic effects through reciprocal connections from the cortex. In this way, a mental sensory loop (Fig. 18a) is formed between the thalamus and cortex, so that the thalamus can more effectively coordinate its incoming hypothalamic effects with previously mapped effects.

When the brain awakens and its physical connections are reestablished, its thalamic loop of mental experience begins to include physical sensory input (Fig. 18b). This inclusion links dream imagery to the perception of physical experience, causing dream recall. Physical experience arouses the prefrontal assessment processes that create long-term memory. Although sensory mapping of mental effects does occur throughout sleep atonia, we do not consciously associate those mental effects with physical experience before the metencephalon arouses and we are again connected to physical reality.

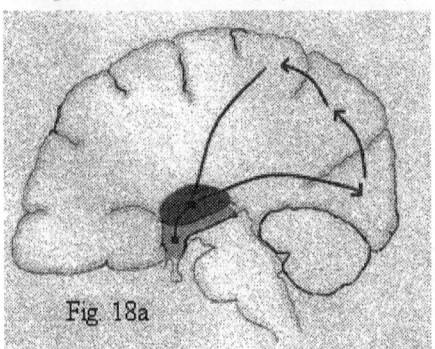

Fig 18a

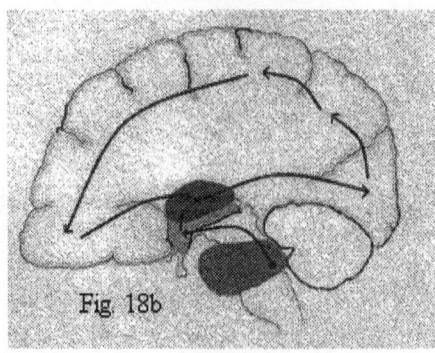

Fig 18b

*   *   *

The brain's reconnection to physical reality will produce memories of dreaming, depending on the dreamer's prefrontal ability to attach material consequences to mental experiences. As we have learned, mental experiences established without physical experience can be difficult to remember. However, some mental experiences can be difficult to forget. Some dreams have curious, sometimes lasting effects on the mind, body, and emotions of the dreamer. In the next chapter, we will explore some of the paradoxes of sleep and dreaming.

REFERENCE

Alavi, A., Dann, R., Chawluk, J., Alavi, J., Kushner, M., and Reivich, M. "Positron Emission Tomography Imaging of Regional Cerebral Glucose Metabolism." *Semin Nucl Med.* (1986): 16(1): 2–34.

Brower, M. C. and Price, B. H. "Neuropsychiatry of Frontal Lobe Dysfunction in Violent and Criminal Behaviour: A Critical Review." *J Neurol Neurosurg Psychiatry* (2001): 71(6): 720–6.

Hong, C. C., Gillin, J. C., Dow, B. M., Wu, J., and Buchsbaum, M.S. "Localized and Lateralized Cerebral Glucose Metabolism Associated with Eye Movements during REM Sleep and Wakefulness: A Positron Emission Tomography (PET) Study." *Sleep* (1995): 8(7): 570–80.

Nolte, J. *The Human Brain: An Introduction to Its Functional Anatomy* (4th ed.). St. Louis: Mosby, 2002.

Owen, A. M., Doyon, J., Petrides, M., and Evans, A.C. "Planning and Spatial Working Memory: A Positron Emission Tomography Study in Humans." *Eur J Neurosci.* (1996): 8(2): 353–64.

Perry, B. D. "Childhood Experiences and the Expression of Genetic Potential: What Childhood Neglect Tells Us about Nature and Nurture." *Brain and Mind* (2002): 3: 79–100.

Wolkin, A., Jaeger, J., Brodie, J. D., Wolf, A. P., Fowler, J., Rotrosen, J., Gomez-Mont, F., and Cancro, R. "Persistence of Cerebral Metabolic Abnormalities in Chronic Schizophrenia as Determined by Positron Emission Tomography. *Am J Psychiatry* (1985): 142(5): 564–71.

There are more things in heaven and earth, Horatio, than are dreamt of in your philosophy.

—William Shakespeare, *Hamlet* (Act I, Scene 5)

CHAPTER VII: Sleep and Dreaming Paradoxes

In previous chapters, we examined the paradoxical nature of the wakefulness occurring in the brain during atonic sleep. By now, we should know that this wakefulness is caused by a physiological adaptation that sustains vital neurological and physiological systems during extended periods of food privation and physical inactivity. We should also know that the neurological effects of this adaptation produce dreaming and restrict gross locomotion. These products have resulted in further paradoxes of mind and body function.

Movement Paradox

Although gross locomotion is restricted when a normal and healthy brain arouses during atonic sleep, smaller movements do occur. These movements are paradoxical to the general nature of sleep atonia. Small movements, such as hand and feet twitching, eye darting, and penile erection, appear to suggest that the brain is not entirely isolated from the musculature of the body and physical experience while dreaming. However, this suggestion is only valid to the extent of the neurological causes of these small movements.

Rapid Eye Movement

Rapid eye movement (REM) is the most recognized physical indicator of dreaming. During REM, visibly darting eye movements beneath closed eyelids signal the onset of dreaming. Although researchers believe they have localized the source of this movement in the metencephalon, the evidence shows that this is not the case. The eye movements researchers have observed in surgically prepared meten-cephalic brains are merely the severed nerve effects that reach the eye musculature during metencephalic dormancy. (See Chapter IV, Preparation Effect/REM.)

In an intact and conscious brain, eye movement begins in the diencephalon through excitation of the superior colliculi (SC). Afferents or inputs to the SC, when the brain is conscious, initiate a cascade of efferent (output) effects from the diencephalon and telencephalon to the musculature of the eye through the metencephalon. When the structures of the diencephalon and telencephalon arouse during metencephalic dormancy, their efferent network of nerves through the metencephalon also arouses. The eye movement we associate with the dream-ing brain is a product of this efferent motor-network arousal. The eye moves while gross body movement is restricted because the musculature of the eye is not controlled by the motor network originating in the metencephalon. Metencephalic dormancy disables its motor network to the body. The control of eye movement by the diencephalic/telencephalic brain also explains why actual tears are produced when dream experiences involve crying.

Twitching

The small spasmodic limb, hand, and foot movements that frequently occur as we drift into sleep and dreaming have obvious associations with the function or dysfunction of the structures in the metencephalon. When metencephalic func-tion is not completely dormant, movement can occur as consciousness moves into sleep and dreaming. Damage or dysfunction of the metencephalon can cause gross movement, such as sleepwalking or "acting out" of dream content. This damage can deceive the brain into perceiving that it is experiencing physical phe-nomena. When conscious, damaged metencephalic function can occlude physi-cal sensory data and cause the brain to perceive mental effects as physical experience.

Sleepwalking

Sleepwalking occurs when the diencephalon and telencephalon have become active during the S-sleep phase of sleep mediated by the metencephalon. Normally, the metencephalon mediates muscle readiness during S-sleep and relinquishes this ready state at the onset of dreaming. When it is functioning abnormally and its control of muscle readiness fails to release, the metencephalon can permit abnormal sleep behavior by allowing tactile sensory data into dream content. This can enable the sensorimotor functions that facilitate sleepwalking.

Damage to the locus ceruleus of the metencephalon has produced such behavior in cats.

Movement and abnormal sleep behavior can also occur through dysfunction in the diencephalon and telencephalon. This can occur when these structures become active before the metencephalon signals its release of muscle readiness. Although not currently understood in this way by researchers, the metencephalon's atonic signals are contained in the impulses issued from its tegmentum (Fig. 14) structure to the hypothalamus at the onset of dreaming. When the diencephalon and telencephalon become prematurely active, the resulting mental activity can produce efferent activity in the musculature of the body before the metencephalon has disabled such activity.

Penile Erection

External to the body, the penis of a normal human male engorges with blood periodically during sleep and dreaming. As a result, the tissues of this organ enter an erect, sexually ready state. This state of sexual readiness during sleep appears to serve no obvious function, since it occurs when males are unable to engage in sexual behavior. Nevertheless, penile erection does serve a physiological function during sleep.

The penis is part of the urogenital system mediated by the hypothalamus. During tonic and atonic sleep, the hypothalamus maintains homeostasis. Although that function is disconnected from the body's musculature by atonia, it remains intact in other vital systems of the body. The penis is linked to those vital systems sustained by the function of the hypothalamus during sleep atonia.

In early animals, external genitalia likely made those organs susceptible to environmental conditions. Consequently, these animals developed a physiology to sustain their external reproductive organs through extended periods of inactivity. Blood flow to the penis brings nutrients and warmth into its structure. The periodic flow of nutrients and warmth into the external organs of early animals would likely have sustained these organs through extended periods of sleep. The penile erection that sleeping human males experience is a physiological vestige of this homeostatic process begun in early animals to sustain their external reproductive organs.

NREM Dreaming Paradox

Some sleep and dream studies appear to provide evidence of dreaming through all phases of sleep. The participants in these studies, through sleep-phase interruptions, have reported dream experiences through some or all of the various stages of sleep preceding dream sleep. Sleep-phase interruptions involve the waking of study participants during each stage of NREM, according to EEG pattern, to assess the occurrence of dreaming. As an investigative tool, phasic interruption of sleep is not a useful or reliable method for assessing dreaming, because it can cause the arousal in the brain that produces dreaming.

We know the brain arouses during metencephalic dormancy. When it arouses prematurely and sleep is interrupted, sensory data from the metencephalon can enter the brain and cause mental effects preceding conscious awareness. These mental effects can accumulate as memory, with a speed equal to that of mental perception. Although dreams may seem to arise through all phases of sleep, NREM dream experiences may merely show the speed at which mental effects become dreams in the awakening brain.

Time-Dilation Paradox

Dreams can transpire within a fragment of normal time. Because dreams are mental experiences, they occur at the speed of brain function. Although some dreams may cause the perception of dilating time, that perception does not reflect the actual speed at which the dreams elapse. The perception of lapsing time is just that: a perception.

Lucid Dreaming

In experiments involving strobe lights placed in proximity to sleeping participants, researchers were able to induce lucid dreaming. Lucid dreaming is the perception of being consciously aware within the unconscious state of dreaming. Researchers have induced this perception of awareness at the onset of REM by flashing proximity lights which study participants previously learned to recognize as a sign that they were experiencing dreams. Visual sensory data, as we have previously learned, enters at the level of brain function and structure above that which isolates the brain from physical sensory data during atonic sleep. Therefore, the sensory from light sources in the sleep environment can enter the brain and become part of dream content, making it identifiable as originating from physical experience. Once this distinction is made—that a dream depiction is originating from physical experience—the dreaming brain is able to detect the distinction between its current state and the state of true physical experience.

Lucid Paralysis

Although dream lucidity can be artificially stimulated, it very often arises naturally and without the introduction of physical sensory data. When this happens, the experience is most commonly accompanied by the dreamer's perception of being in bed or lying down and unable to move. Dreamers have reported secondary perceptions of deafening white noise, feeling weighted down, bed tremors, and dark figures moving about the sleep environment while the dreamer remains paralyzed. The paralysis, weightiness, and white noise are explainable through the brain's loss of sensory contact through metencephalic dormancy. These physical sensations and sounds are how the wakeful diencephalic/telencephalic brain interprets the mental effects caused by its detection of metencephalic inactivity.

The higher brain's efferent motor network coordinates its function through the motor network arising in the metencephalon. The brain uses the metencephalon's network to execute muscle commands. When the metencephalon becomes inactive, its motor network is disabled. The perceived absence of motor afferents (feedback) to the brain from its motor efferents (commands) to the musculature during a dream probably causes the mental effects leading to the lucid perception of paralysis. The accompanying bed tremors and bedroom intruders manifest the mental effects of the fear caused by the perception of being unable to move.

Whether artificially induced or transpiring as paralysis, lucidity can occur at any moment and manifest a sense of conscious experience whenever a dreamer, while dreaming, becomes cognizant of the distinction between the dream and true physical experience. This distinction denotes the arousal of prefrontal activity and its assessment of a mental experience as consequential to true physical experience.

Metaphysical Paradox

Lucid dreaming, religious imagery, precognition, telepathy, telekinesis, out-of-body experiences (OBE), and after-death contact with the deceased are several of the dream experiences many dreamers report as having some lasting effect on their conscious thoughts, feelings, and actions. In earlier chapters, we learned how Jung was profoundly influenced by imagery of God in his dream and how Lincoln was said to have foreseen his own assassination in a dream. These wondrous and uncanny experiences appear to defy rational explanation. However, a basis in brain function and structure for these experiences must exist, because nothing can arise in the brain without such a basis.

After-Death Contact (ADC)

Lucid dreaming has its basis in the brain's ability to distinguish the mental experience of dreaming from true physical experience. This can be accomplished artificially through the introduction of physical sensory data outside the dream state, or it can arise naturally through the normal course of dreaming. A type of lucid dream experience is the recognition, while dreaming, of a deceased person in a dream.

Contact with the deceased during a dream is a common occurrence. Usually, the dreamer does not recognize the person as deceased until he awakens from the dream and recalls the event of that person's demise. Sometimes the dreamer recognizes the deceased person's status and become lucidly aware of his own status within a dream. Such lucid experiences usually lead to arousal from sleep. However, other dreams of deceased persons occur when the dreamers could not possibly know that those persons are deceased. These dreams present in a manner that seems more lucid than physical reality. Also, they appear to arise at nearly the moment of the deceased person's death. Consider the following dream:

> One night in May '97, I dreamed he was tapping on my window like he had always done when he wanted me to come outside. "Shave and a haircut, two bits." I ran outside (it was night in my dream) and greeted him. He looked as he did in the last picture I had of him. I didn't bother to ask why he was there, because he began asking me questions. I told him pretty much everything that was going on in my life. Then I finally asked him why he was in town, and he only responded by smiling. Then he pointed at a star and said, "Remember that star." Then he kissed me on the cheek, like he did when I last saw him, and disappeared. I woke up, wondering what it was all about, thinking it was because I would be visiting him in a few weeks and because we always used to go out and stargaze as little kids. But a week later, his parents sent me a letter saying he had been killed in a car crash on the same night I had the dream. I haven't told anybody about that dream, because I'm afraid they'd say I made it up. But it did happen, and I have thought about it every day since I heard of his death.

The dreamer said that she experienced this dream when she was sixteen and that it involved a close childhood friend who moved out of state when they were both several years younger. She said they had maintained contact through the years and that she had planned to visit him that summer. A cogent argument could be made for the dreamer's initial belief that her dream was merely a product of the lingering mental effects of planning and anticipating a visit to a dear friend. However, the imagery in her dream suggests otherwise, because dream imagery does not translate as something the dreamer would literally experience.

Dream imagery translates mental effects; therefore, the above dream references the mental impact of her friendship with the person depicted. What make this dream a true after-death contact (ADC) experience is provided by its translation and emphasized by its depiction of her friend's behavior. In that depiction, we observe typical ADC behaviors that can include the decedent's reticence, the absence of perceived physical contact except that initiated by the decedent, and the decedent's avoidance of questions. Upon waking from such experiences, the dreamer is usually confused about the nature and significance of the encounter, because it appears more lucid than true physical experience. When a dreamer discovers the reality of the person's death, she immediately recalls their dream encounter and is reluctant to discuss it. The possibility of ADC has a theoretical basis in what might make telepathy possible.

Telepathy

The possibility that the human brain may be capable of perceiving thoughts and other information ethereally has been the object of some serious study over the years. It was studied by Dr. J. B. Rhine in his parapsychology laboratory at Duke University and studied by the CIA and the KGB in secret experiments to determine the practical application of telepathy to covert intelligence. However, serious interest does not prove the brain's capacity to detect ethereal sensory data. If the brain is capable of detecting this kind of sensory data, a basis must exist in brain structure and function.

We can find many examples of animals whose sensory acuity exceeds human capability. They can see farther than us and in pitch-darkness, they can hear sounds at higher and lower frequencies, and they can smell blood in the ocean or taste prey in the air several miles farther away. The sensory systems of some animals are more highly developed than ours. Accordingly, their cortices are able to receive and map sensory information that our brains cannot detect. The evidence suggests that human ancestors relinquished much of their sensory acuity for the capacity to think and reason beyond the ability of other animals. This has allowed us to become the dominant species despite our sensory shortfall. For the moment, consider the implication of the human brain's evolution beyond the physical senses thus far.

Over several million years, the human brain evolved to receive and map sensory information in ways that have placed our species above others whose survival advantage would be greater if we had only our senses on which to rely. Among the abilities of autistic savants, we find evidence of the human brain's capacity to map information in ways that produce astonishing results.

The extraordinary potential of the human brain is mirrored in the savant capacity to play concertos without receiving music lessons, to sculpt and paint masterpieces without lessons in art, and to remember statistical information for several years in incredible detail. Daniel Tammet, a savant billed as "Brain Man," performs intricate and lengthy math computations mentally in a fraction of the time required by others of average brain function. He speaks several languages and can learn a new language in about a week just by hearing others speak it. Insight into these remarkable mental abilities may reside in his memory function.

In an interview on his remarkable math ability, Daniel described an emotional connection to numbers. He said that each number felt different, presenting as a nebulous form in his mind's eye. When performing large computations in multi-plication, each multiplier appears in his mind as a separate mass, and the solution arises between them as another mass. Although researchers do not fully under-stand his phenomenal mental abilities, Daniel's emotional connection with num-bers and their nebulous forms suggest the considerable contributions of his amygdala and hippocampus to his extraordinary brain function.

As we know, the significance of the amygdala and the hippocampus to mem-ory is considerable. The way Daniel's brain coordinates and maps the visual sen-sory information of numbers with the memory functions of these structures plausibly produces the emotional effects, anomalous forms, and extended mem-ory necessary to his math computations. Succinctly, his brain maps common sen-sory data in ways that produce uncommon results.

The brain's ability to produce uncommon results from common sensory data theoretically supports the general nature of telepathy. Knowing what a person might be thinking or feeling through behavioral observations is common. Theoretically, common behavioral observations might become much more under the right mental conditions. Those conditions might present while we are con-scious, through autism, or while we sleep, through dreaming. In its isolation from physical experience, the dreaming brain could theoretically become telepathic.

Precognition

Precognitive dreams translate the mental effects of experiences the dreamer may subsequently encounter in physical reality. Unlike psychic precognition, precog-nitive dreams do not involve literal depictions of future occurrences; they depict the mental effects of perceived future experiences. The possibility of precognition in dream content is supported by the savant effect of sensory isolation. In such isolation, resonant mental effects could be coordinated and mapped in ways similar to Daniel Tammet's math ability. Theoretically, a dreamer could experience separate mental effects that combine in dream content to produce imagery suggestive of future effects.

Miscellaneous Phenomena

All dream phenomena, no matter how wondrous, define the sense of something that has had an affect on the dreamer's unconscious mind. Phenomena like lucid dreams, after-death contact, telepathy, and precognition all describe how the brain perceives it has been mentally affected by some influence or influences. Therefore, every experience in dream content should be understood from the perspective of the perceptions they translate. For example, out-of-body experiences translate the perception or mental sense of leaving or abandoning one's earthly identity or nature; telekinesis translates the sense of mastery over perception or perceived influences; telepathy translates the perception of precisely understanding what others may think or feel; and lucid dreaming translates the perception of understanding the reality of one's situation. Dreams resembling these phenomena express the profound mental effects caused by the resonant effects of life experiences.

Religious and Spiritual Imagery

We have nearly reached the end of the journey we began several chapters ago. Some of us may have begun this journey inspired by dreams similar to Dr. Jung's. Some may believe that if messages from a supreme being or supreme consciousness are possible, they will come as dreams. Spirituality and faith have a powerful impact on our psychology and the dream content that psychology kindles. Although dreams reflect the mental impact of our beliefs, they do not necessarily validate those beliefs. Dreams do not translate literal truths; they translate the mental effects of what we believe to be truth. Therefore, our dreams can elaborate the leading or misleading mental effects of our beliefs.

*   *   *

The paradoxes of sleep and dreaming can distort our conclusions about their nature and their significance to our conscious experience. Our only guard against the probability of self-deception through misperception is to continuously examine the basis for them as new evidence emerges. Although much of the evidence we have examined is not new, we may now perceive it in a new way. In the next chapter, we will attempt to define a clearer and more personally relevant path to translating the implications of specific dream imagery and content.

REFERENCE

LaBerge, S. "Lucid Dreaming: Psychophysiological Studies of Consciousness during REM Sleep," in R. R. Bootzen, J. F. Kihlstrom, and D. L. Schacter (eds.), *Sleep and Cognition*. Washington: APA, 1990.

Parker, A. and Brusewitz, G. "A Compendium of the Evidence for Psi." *European Journal of Parapsychology* (2003): 18: 33–51.

Shouse, M. N. and Siegel, J. M. "Pontine Regulation of REM Sleep Components in Cats: Integrity of the Pedunculopontine Tegmentum (PPT) Is Important for Phasic Events but Unnecessary for Atonia during REM Sleep." *Brain Res.* (1992): 571: 50–63.

Enlightenment isn't how much you know about the world or whether you know the secrets of the universe; it's how much you know about yourself and your reason for being.

—The author

CHAPTER VIII: Translation

Interpretation is an inadequate description for the psychologically useful form of dream imagery. It erroneously implies that the meaning of imagery varies from dreamer to dreamer; it implies that a house as mental shelter in one person's dream may suggest the body in someone else's. Dreams are distinctly mental in origin, nature, and substance. The certainty of their mental quality assures us that every influence perceived while dreaming collectively describes something mental and something of mental impact. Houses will always translate as the effects of mental structures in dreams. Rather than "interpretation," "translation" is more descriptive of this well-defined process of relating dream imagery to mental influence.

Sensory Spawn

Everything about brain structure and function tells us that its development and corollary activity are products of afferent sensory information. Perhaps beginning in a cluster of photosensitive epidermal cells, for example, light stimulated the growth of these cells into surrounding tissues, producing a photosensitive neural network that progressed into other structures and spawned diencephalic development in the primitive brain. All brain structures, from the myelencephalon to the telencephalon, followed this sense-led path to developments that progressively enhanced brain function and provided survival advantages.

Following the senses, each new level of brain structure owes its origin and function to the behaviors and advantages birthed by the sensory perceptions of preceding levels. The metencephalon owes its development to the myelencephalon; the diencephalon is indebted to metencephalic/myelencephalic function; and the telencephalon owes its existence to the functions of the diencephalic/meten-cephalic/myelencephalic structure. This pattern of brain evolution, ascending from its most primitive structure, explains why the isolation of the cortex by surgical transaction produces a continuous state of slow-wave activity.

Subcortical Significance

In animal experiments, isolation of the cortex from the brain's substructures produced continuous slow-wave activity in the cortex. Because this structure's development and function are dependent on those of the brain structures preceding it, cortical activity will remain dormant whenever the cortex is rendered incapable of receiving input from those substructures. Therefore, no product of cortical activity, including dream content, is possible without input from subcortical structures. If an electrochemical disturbance in brain function arises in the cortex, it is a response to subcortical inputs.

Cortical Implications

Consider, with dreaming aside for the moment, the substantial implication of brain function suggested by the ineffectiveness of the cortex without its substructures. Essentially, the hierarchy of brain development and function—manifesting human consciousness and all that we know ourselves to be—does not descend from the cortex; it ascends from the brainstem through the cortex. The cortex controls and initiates nothing, not even its own activity, without directives from subcortical structures. When aberrant behaviors manifest through abnormalities of the cortex, they reflect how subcortical directives can be skewed by distorted paths through the cortex. Indeed, the implication is that the cortex is nothing more than a map or the working space through which subcortical functions are attenuated and executed. When parts of the cortex are damaged, it merely constructs new maps, tracing different paths to the objectives of subcortical directives. This explains why some cortical damage does not endanger life, and why so much of normal brain function rebounds afterwards.

Dreaming

Dreaming results in the isolation of the diencephalon and telencephalon from the senses and musculature mediated by other substructures. It begins when the tegmentum, a structure of the metencephalon, electrochemically signals metencephalic dormancy to the hypothalamus. The ensuing electrochemical disturbance effects dreaming and energy uptake by the brain and other vital systems during the extended period of physical inactivity characterized by muscle atonia.

The electrochemical disturbance of atonic sleep causes mental effects rippling from the hypothalamus through the thalamus and into the cortex, where a mental loop is formed between it and the thalamus. Physical experience enters the loop and encodes its content with markers that become dream recall when metencephalic function arouses the brain to conscious experience.

The markers of physical experience that become dream recall identify the mental effects experienced by the brain after the electrochemical disturbance initiated in the hypothalamus by the tegmentum. Put more succinctly, dreams describe mental effects. The surrealism of dreams makes translating the effects they describe dauntingly difficult. However, they do follow some rules of logic and reason. In translating your own dream experiences, here are several steps you should consider:

Step 1

Forget everything you have learned about dreaming from all sources other than what you discover through this book. All other works on dreaming are tainted by inadequate or flawed investigatory tools, methods, and assumptions. Adhering to other ideas will only cause you confusion.

Step 2

Every experience and perception in a dream describes something that has influenced you mentally. Therefore, you should discount the physical appearances of your dreams and perceive each aspect of them as a mental affect. If it will help, write out your dream and prefix every description with the word "mental":

> ***Mentally**, I **mentally** went to the **mental** bathroom to **mentally** wash my **mental** hands with **mental** soap and **mentally** saw my*

> *mental reflection in the **mental** mirror **mentally** above the **mental** washbasin.*

No matter how extraordinary you find your dream content, consider it first and foremost as suggestive of mental influences, rather than of actual physical experience.

Step 3

See your dream-self as your consciousness and everything else as something that has influenced your consciousness. In the above example, "I" describes the awareness of the dreamer, and everything else describes something that has reached that awareness.

Step 4

The mental effects your dreams describe follow the sequence of your dream recall, so you should begin to think about the mental distinction of your dream content from the beginning of your description. Using the above example, think about what "Mentally, I" means, then write it down. Next to it, write down what "mentally went" means, and so on with the remainder of your dream content. Near the end of this chapter, I have included an imagery dictionary to assist you with your translations.

Step 5

After writing out your translation, see if it has an intelligible or congruent flow. Abrupt changes in dream imagery very often signify a change in the nature of the thoughts suggested by dream content. This is like thinking about one thing while being reminded of another.

Step 6

If you are satisfied with the congruity of your translation, search your recent experiences or the experiences of the people in your life for the resonant life experience or experiences that likely caused your dream. It is important that you do this after your dream translation, so as not to prejudice your perspective with preconceived opinions.

Should you remain uncertain of your dream's meaning or cause after following the steps I have given, do not be discouraged. The more practiced you become at translating your dreams, the better you will surely become at understanding their content.

IMAGERY DICTIONARY

Everything in dreams is suggestive of something that has some mental effect. Every influence and how you experience each influence within a dream is potentially meaningful; it would not be part of your dream otherwise. The faux sensory experiences of sight, sound, scent, touch, and taste within dreams are particularly suggestive of the type of impact a mental influence has had on your consciousness.

SENSORY IMAGERY

In dreams, the dreamer is representative of the primary mental qualities that render awareness. Those qualities are the capacity to perceive and distinguish influences and the capacity to be affected by influences. The aspect of your awareness that is capable of perceiving and distinguishing influences we shall call insight. We shall call the other aspect your psyche. Together, insight and psyche make up the essence of what you describe within a dream. The sensory experiences you recall from dream content describes how you believe your insight and psyche have been impacted by the influences reverberating in your mind, during atonia, from conscious experience.

Sight (Insubstantial Impact)

Compare to other faux sensory experiences within a dream, what you perceive by sight is the least meaningful. Visual imagery, when it is not accompanied by any other sensory experience, implies a superficial quality of perception, understanding, and mental impact. It suggests that the mental influences described visually in your dream are something you perceive as apparent, self-evident, or easy to understand. Although you may not understand the surreal experiences of your dreams, their visual imagery suggests that their translated effects would be simple to understand.

Sound (Resonant Impact)

Each sensory experience, in the context of dreaming, suggests a different aspect of the way your unconscious mind perceives and understands the mental influences arousing its activity. Sound imagery suggests your perception and understanding of resonance. When mental effects and influences manifest as sound in your dreams, they suggest your perception of some relevance or meaning beyond what may be apparent. In this way, what you hear is more meaningful than what you see in a dream.

Scent (Ambient Impact)

Scent experiences describe your perception of the ambience or mood suggested by the mental circumstances of the life experiences resonant in dream content. For example, the scent of bug spray describes the mental ambience or social mood associated with eliminating pesky mental afflictions.

Touch (Substantial Impact)

Tactile dream sensations are the most meaningful experiences, because they suggest those mental effects and influences that substantially impact your psyche. Any experience, whether or not you are the initiator, involving faux physical contact with any part of your body in a dream describes something that has had a palpable affect on some aspect of your mental being. These dream experiences describe your sense of the mental connection that has transpired between you and a suggested influence that is distinctly apart from what you perceive yourself to be. If contact is made but not felt, then no mental connection of real consequence has occurred, although superficially it may appear otherwise.

Taste (Experiential Impact)

Anything you taste or eat in a dream has some relevance to what you may or may not find inwardly satisfying or meaningful. In conscious reality, tasting is often a prelude to eating. We eat to satisfy our hunger or cravings. The imagery with which you have oral contact describes how you satisfy your inner yearnings.

DIRECTIONAL IMAGERY

The directional perspectives we take for granted in conscious reality are as meaningful as all other imagery in the context of a dream. The placement of imagery relative to your position in a dream describes your perspective of the source, within your mental purview, of the influences that reach your unconscious mental awareness.

Front

Generally, the imagery you experience directly in front of you describes perceptions that have reached your awareness through foresight. When you approach this imagery through your own effort, this describes the foresight you have gained through your independent effort. When the imagery approaches you, as in clouds arriving from a distance, this describes your foresight of influences that may eventually have some impact on your awareness that you may encounter without any effort of your own.

In a twist of frontal meaning, the frontal aspects of the imagery you experience describe the direct aspects of the mental influences they suggest. For example, the front of a house describes what you perceive as the direct aspect of some mental or social structure or experience. Approaching a dream image from its front suggests your approach to a direct aspect of the mental effects or influences it reflects.

Rear

The opposite of the imagery in front of you in a dream is the imagery you perceive behind you. Imagery to your rear describes your perception of the mental effects and influences you experience in hindsight or through retrospection. However, to perceive the rear of a dream image is to perceive the indirect aspects of its suggested effects and influences. Your approach to the rear of imagery describes your approach to some indirect aspect of a suggested mental influence.

Right

Interestingly, imagery positioned to the right of you describes the mental effects and influences you perceive through direct evidence. These are effects and influences upon your insight and psyche that reach your awareness through what you have directly experienced. The implication of right-positioned imagery suggests what you know to be clear, certain, and specific.

Left

Imagery to your left suggests the perceptions that reach your awareness indirectly. This imagery describes those influences you perceive as not based on anything specific. As an indication of the influences affecting your unconscious mind, imagery to your left is less reliable than the imagery to your right. Dream imagery to your left suggests what you perceive without any basis in real or direct evidence.

Right *vs.* Left

The variations in meaning suggested by right and left imagery are tied to the function of the right and left hemispheres of the brain. Currently, science has designated distinct functions for each hemisphere, based on the deficits researchers have found when either side is damaged. According to current scientific thought, brain function is not symmetrical; *e.g.,* language processing is a function of the right hemisphere, while math is a primary function of the left. In fact, the evolutionary evidence suggests that there is symmetry of brain function, only not in the way scientists currently understand.

The human brain has evolved to process sensory information from two perspectives: subjective and objective. The distinction between these two perspectives is akin to what you perceive about yourself as opposed to what you perceive about yourself based on the responses of other people. Language is processed primarily in the right hemisphere because it is more responsive to objective or abstract sensory information: perceptions gathered indirectly. Math is processed primarily in the left hemisphere because it reacts more to subjective or direct sensory experience: perceptions based on personal experience and practical application. The implications of left and right brain function are reversed in dream content, with right imagery suggesting subjective influences and left suggesting objective, because that is how the influences that effect dreaming initially enter the structures of the brainstem that precipitates dreaming.

TRANSLATIONS

The following imagery translations should be considered from the perspective of action relative to you. For example, the translation for "cat" can describe some aspect of your behavior, how you perceive the behavior of some other person, or how you perceive some general nature of human behavior. The distinction between these three could be determined respectively by whether the cat is yours in the dream, whether it belongs to someone else, or whether it belongs to no one. Furthermore, ownership of this animal in your dream may not always describe how you perceive some aspect of your behavior, if you have children. In this instance, your cat may suggest how you perceive the behavior of your children or child. Likewise, when the cat belongs to a friend who has children in real life, it could suggest how you perceive the children of that friend. Further still, if you actually own the cat in reality, it almost certainly suggests how you perceive some quality of that specific animal. Anything you perceive in dream content as belonging to you probably describes the mental influence of something you perceive as directly related to or associated with you. What does not belong to you in a dream describes effects and influences from sources beyond yourself.

Mental *vs.* Social

Generally, the influences that sway your mind also affect your social perspective. For this reason, you may also prefix dream imagery with the word "social." The image of a house, for example, can describe either a mental or a social structure. I realize how confusing this must be. However, translating dream imagery is rarely a simple process, even for those as experienced as myself. As a rule, whatever involves your dream persona's actions and tactile perceptions suggests something distinctly mental. Otherwise, something distinctly social is suggested. Running imagery, for example, describes a mental effort when you are the person engaging this activity. Conversely, a social effort is suggested when you dream of seeing other people running.

*   *   *

With the following list of translations, you have reached the end of the journey you began several chapters ago. It is my hope that you have learned something about the nature of mind, consciousness, and dreaming (beyond the psychological and neurological dogma of the past 100 years) that has inspired a more enlightened perspective of your mental nature. Through several decades of studying dreams and dreaming, I have learned how little we truly understand about ourselves. Despite our technologies, we are a primitive species whose baser aspects exert a potent influence over our being. When we begin to understand the true nature of our dreams, we begin to breakdown the mental barriers within us that could cause mental dysfunction and misdeed. As you pursue your dream studies, you will discover that dreams are truly thoughts manifested as physical experiences. Although they are mental phenomena, you will find that your dreams are every bit as significant as your experiences in the physical world; they have impact of profound significance to your mental and social well-being. Considering your dreams with the same regard as your physical experiences will enhance the quality of your life. Sleep well.

ENTRIES: A-Z

A

accident: An incident of mental or social impact; an unintended or unexpected incident.

acting: Uncharacteristic social attitude or behavior.

activity: Mental or social responses to mental or social influences.

address: The position of a mental or social structure; situation of a mental or social experience.

advertisement: An attempt to gain mental or social attention or recognition.

AIDS: A debilitating and wretched state of mind and emotion probably caused by a failed or tragic intimate relationship. (See **sexual disease**.)

aiming: Focused; goal or objective-oriented.

air conditioning: Clearing the air figuratively; calming mental or social tensions.

airplane: Mental or social aspirations; lofty ambitions, pursuits, endeavors, or expectations.

airplane crash: Failure of mental or social aspirations. (See **airplane**.)

algebra: Rational or logical applications or associations; reasoning. (See **math** and **numbers**.)

alien: A personage of uncommon or extraordinary mental perception, experience, or ability; mental or social perceptions beyond the mundane, terrestrial, or ordinary; the perception of unearthly mental or social influences; mental or social influence without basis in reality.

alligator: (See **crocodile**.)

ambulance: A medical urgency.

American Indian: Fundamentalist; a personage of fundamental mental and social perception; fundamental perceptions. (Note: The translations provided are not reflective of the true and noble nature of these people. These are merely subliminal distinctions based on the primitive, often uncivil way humanity perceives its own. Racial imagery in dream content describes our perception of a class or social distinction. The translations here may only apply to imagery in the dreams of non-American Indians.)

angel: A personage of celestial, divine, or metaphysical mental or social influence.

animals: Instinctive attitudes and behaviors; instinctive, ignoble aspects of human nature; mental or social influences arising from physical drives and nature. (See **ape, armadillo, bear, bird, cat, chicken, crocodile, dog, fox,**

groundhog, horse, lion, mouse, monkey, pig, rat, shark, skunk, snake, stuffed animals, wildcat, and wolf.)

ants: Trivial annoyances; insanity. (See **insects**.)

ape: Social or intellectual primitive; brutish, unenlightened nature. (See **animals**.)

apparel: (See **clothes**.)

applause: Approval.

armadillo: Obstinacy; intractable nature. (See **animals**.)

arrival: The conclusion of mental or social journey.

Asian: An industrious personage; industrious mental or social influence. (Note: The translations provided are not reflective of the true and noble nature of these people. These are merely subliminal distinctions based on the primitive, often uncivil way humanity perceives its own. Racial imagery in dream content describes our perception of a class or social distinction. The translations here may only apply to imagery in the dreams of non-Asians.)

audience: Mass social interests or attention; a like-minded collective.

auditorium: A mental or social environment or experience in which public interest or attention is amassed.

award: A recognition of accomplishment.

ax: A mental or social means by which an influence could be rendered asunder; a means to cause traumatic division.

B

baby: A social bond; a suggestion of that which requires mental or social nurturing; a new mental or social awareness.

back door: An alternative or indirect access; an indirect access to a social structure or experience; an indirect access to a mental structure or experience.

back pain: The lingering mental or emotional pain or discomfort associated with a memory.

bandit: One who takes unfair advantage of others. (See **burglar**.)

bank: An income-associated environment or experience.

bank check: Conditional income; income dependent on the settlement or outcome of circumstances; potential gain.

baseball: A mental or social game that is slow and deliberate. (See **game**.)

basement: A lower mental or social standard; a lower standard of living.

bath: A cleansing of conscience; mental cleansing.

bathroom: A cleansing experience; an experience associated with purging rancor, frustration, and sin. (See **defecation, feces, restroom, toilet, urination,** and **urine.**)

bathtub: The activity within a cleansing experience associated with regaining self-respect.

beach: A lack of firm mental or social foundation; threshold to a potentially meaningful social experience. (See **ground.**)

bear: Overbearing, domineering nature. (See **animals.**)

bed: Intimate activity; intimate activity associated with creating social bonds and restoring vitality.

beer: A delusional mental or social influence; a meaningful experience with delusional mental or social effects.

bees: Stinging, irritating, or aggravating mental or social influence. (See **insects.**)

bicycle: An activity associated with mental balance.

birds: Flightiness; free-spiritedness. (See **animals.**)

birdcage: That which confines a free spirit. (See **birds.**)

birth: Emergence of a new social bond; emergence of an affecting and effective social or mental influence; emergence of a new social awareness.

black: Mystique; an indefinable distinction; mystery; foreboding. (See **darkness,** and **night.**)

blackheads: (See **pimples.**)

blanket: An enveloping influence that may either conceal or comfort.

blind: The incapacity to perceive what should be clear and apparent to anyone. (See **eyes.**)

blood: Vitality.

blue: Calm; serenity.

boat: A mental or social vessel of transport across the fluid conditions of life experience; prosperity.

bomb: A potentially explosive mental or social influence; a socially explosive incident; a non-constructive incident with personal repercussions.

book: An embodiment of specific knowledge or insight.

boss: The compelling mental or social influence associated with responsibility and obligation.

box: A finite or limited perspective; a conscious conclusion.

brain: Intelligence.

breakfast: A meaningful or inwardly satisfying experience that comes after a lengthy period of uncertainty and self-denial.

breast: Exposure of vulnerability, sensitivity, and trust.

bridge: A mental or social transition; an association.

building: A depiction of the mental or social structure associated with the type of building; an environment of social routine and diversity associated with the business of life.

buried: Overwhelmed; denigrated; concealed.

burglar: A social intruder. (See **bandit**.)

burn: Mental or social disdain; to spurn.

butler: A personage of subservience to the privileged.

C

cancer: Although not imminent, a reference to the inevitability of death.

candle: Archaic source of insight or enlightenment.

candy: A sweet or delightful mental or social indulgence.

canyon: (See **chasm**.)

car: A mental or social vehicle; mental or social drive.

carnival: A serious social incident or experience treated with frivolous disregard; carnival-like social circumstance.

cat: Vanity; snobbery; diva-like social behavior. (See **animals**.)

Catholic: Suggestive of mainstream religion; religious tradition.

chair: A fixed mental or social perspective; a position of thought.

chasm: A mental or social divide; a mental or social rift.

chased: Tormented; menaced.

chess: Patience, planning, and focus. (See **game**.)

chicken: Skittishness; unreasonable fear. (See **animals**.)

child: Immaturity; naiveté; inexperience; social bond.

Christmas: Period of youthful anticipation; a new spiritual beginning.

church: Spiritual or religious structure; spiritual or religious experience.

cigarette: A habit or obsession; a detrimental habit.

circle: A mental or social cycle.

circus: (See **carnival**.)

city: Sense of one's place in society; a social collective.

classroom: A learning experience.

climbing: A effort to reach some mental or social pinnacle.

clock: Time; timing.

closet: Secrets; concealment.

clothed: Mentally or socially prepared; pretentious.

clothes: Social images; self-perceptions that conceal one's true nature or vulnerabilities; pretensions.

clouds: Omens; fantasy; whimsy; dreams.

clown: Foolishness; buffoonery; silliness.

cockroach: Disease; pestilence; perception of unsanitary influences. (See **insects**.)

coffin: Corporeal death; deathlike experience.

cold: Devoid of social warmth.

college: A higher level of learning; formal preparation for some task. (See **school**.)

computer: The mechanism of mind and reason.

concrete: Reliable; mentally or socially firm; substantial.

cookies: Mental or social treats; delightful indulgences.

cooking: The process of preparing an inwardly satisfying experience; an effort to render a meaningful experience more palatable.

costume: Façade.

cousin: Kinship; an affinity felt for another.

cracks: Imperfections; mistakes; incompleteness.

crime: Injustice.

crocodile: Subversiveness. (See **animals**.)

crossroads: Convergent or divergent mental or social paths.

crying: (See **tears**.)

cup: A source of some potentially meaningful or inwardly satisfying perception.

D

dancing: A harmonious effort.

darkness: Ignorance; fear. (See **night**.)

daylight: Enlightened mental or social perspective; optimism; positive social climate, period, or interval.

dead: Apathetic; disillusioned; ineffectual; dispirited. (See **death** and **dying**.)

deaf: Incapable of perceiving or understanding more than the superficial or apparent; a lack of in-depth perception or insight.

death: The perception of an irretrievable mental or social loss. (See **dead** and **dying**.)

defecation: An expression or release of rancor; a rancorous release or expression of some pent-up feeling. (See **bathroom**, **feces**, **restroom**, and **toilet**.)

demon: A manifestation of fear and ignorance; a character flaw.

desert: Mental or social desolation.

dessert: A delightful indulgence or distraction associated with a truly meaningful experience.

devil: Temptation.

dinosaurs: Archaic, primal behavior that has no place in modern society. (See **animals.**)

dirt: Sin; aspersion; degradation.

dirty: disreputable; foul; scurrilous; sinful.

disease: An unhealthy mental or social state. (See **AIDS** and **sexual disease.**)

doctor: A social influence perceived as knowledgeable in the treatment of mental and social illnesses.

dog: Loyalty; obedience; a representation of the behavior associated with basic human nature. (See **animals.**)

dog bark: Social warning associated with faithful companionship.

dog bite: Ingratitude.

door: Opportunity; a mental or social access.

driving: Self-motivated.

drunk: Delusional; a lack of self-discipline; deleterious overindulgence.

dying: A mental decline; a decline in effectiveness or relevance; the inclination of disaffection. (See **dead** and **death.**)

E

ear: Depth of perception; an indication of the capacity or ability to comprehend beyond the superficial or apparent. (See **deaf.**)

Earth: Terrestrial; reality; a reference to physical reality.

earthquake: A traumatic mental or social adjustment.

eggs: Fragility; faith.

elderly: Experienced; wise; archaic or traditional social influence.

electricity: Inspiration; mental or emotional shock.

elevator: An experience controlled by fate or faith.

embrace: Acceptance; trust; love.

eruption: Social upheaval.

eyes: Awareness; an indication of the capacity or ability to comprehend that which is apparent or self-evident; paranoia.

F

face: Personality; identity.

faceless: Without personality or identity; a representation of not truly knowing another.

face slap: An affront.

fall: Failure; a failure to maintain a prior mental or social position or level.

falling objects from clouds: Premonitions; nebulous influences of real and probable impact.

falling objects to earth: Influences of real impact on life. (See **Earth**.)

fat: (See **obese**.)

father: Provider; a personage concerned with the support and protection of the vulnerable.

fear: Inadequacy.

feces: Rancor; disgust. (See **bathroom**, **defecation**, and **restroom**.)

feet: Sense of self associated with self-assurance.

female: A receptive mental or social influence; a feminine influence.

fence: Social mores and barriers.

fight: Antagonism. (See **war**.)

fire: Persecution.

fish: Meaningful opportunity or venture.

flag: Symbolism.

floor: Mental or social foundation. (See **ground**.)

flying: (See **levitation**.)

forest: Mental or social obstructions to a clearer perspective.

fox: Opportunistic nature or behavior. (See **animals**.)

fruit: A meaningful result of growth and experience.

G

gambling: A representation of risk-taking.

game: The healthy give and take, confrontation, and competitiveness of life experience. (See **baseball** and **chess**.)

garbage: Inconsequential.

gay: (See **homosexual**.)

genitalia: A reference to sexual identity, awareness, or interest.

ghost: A lingering social influence or perception.

giants: Exaggeration; imposing or intimidating mental or social influences.

gold: Intrinsic mental or social value or worth.

grandparents: Traditional social guidance or wisdom; traditional social values.

ground: Foundation; basis; a basis in reality.

groundhog: Skeptic; subversion of basis; undermining. (See **animals**.)

gun: Offensiveness; aggression; perceptions capable of inflicting penetrating mental or emotional wounds.

H

hair: Thought; a perception of thought.
hairless: Thoughtless. (See **skinhead**.)
hammer: Forceful perceptions.
handcuffed: Controlled; an inability to act freely.
hands: Ability; mental grasp, control, or perception; sense of personal ease.
hats: Fixed mental attitude.
home: Socially secure; stability.
homeless: Social insecurity or instability.
homosexual: A personage with an emotional dislike for the opposite sex.
horse: A noble aspect of human nature or behavior. (See **animals**.)
hospital: A structured healing experience.
house: A mental or social structure; an environment of structured mental and social experience. (See **building** and **home**.)

I

ice cream: A delightful indulgence that is devoid of emotional warmth.
injury: A mental or emotional hurt or wound.

insects: Trivial annoyances; unnerving perceptions; pestilence. (See **bees** and **cockroach**.)

K

kill: To render ineffective; to eradicate mentally or socially. (See **dead**, **death**, and **dying**.)
king: An ultimate authority.
kiss: Sincere affection.
knife: Divisive or incisive perceptions.

L

legs: A reference to self-confidence.
levitation: Mentally liberated from worldly concerns.
library: A perceived repository of collective knowledge.

light: Enlightenment; mental illumination; clarity.
lion: Proud nature or behavior; defensiveness. (See **animals**.)

M

male: An masculine mental or social influence.
marriage: A social commitment.
math: An analytical process.
medicine: A mental or social remedy.
military: A reference to social order; oppression; a perspective of the social establishment.
money: Perceptions associated with the influence of mental or social worth.
monkey: A perception of disruptive, uncivil nature or behavior. (See **animals**.)
monster: A perception of mental or social ugliness.
moon: An inspiring or enlightened perception during a period of social uncertainty, pessimism, or fear. (See **night**.)
mother: Nurture; a personage of unconditional love and devotion.
mountain: A monumental or lofty challenge; a monumental endeavor; a lofty impediment.
mouse: A perception of scurrilous nature; flirtatiousness. (See **animals** and **rat**.)
mud: Convolution; degradation. (See **dirt** and **dirty**.)
music: A harmonious mental perception.

N

naked: (See **nude**.)
name: A perception of identity; a perception of possessing a means to recognize or identity some mental or social influence.
neighbor: A social peer or competitor.
night: A period of forebode or uncertain; a period of social misfortune; a pessimistic social perspective.
nude: A perception of intimate or personal exposure or vulnerability; unpreparedness; immodesty; unpretentiousness; uninhibited.
number: A perception of that which is both basic and abstract.

O

obese: A perception of overindulgence; a personage of excessive carnal gratification.
ocean: A perception of the vast expanse of life's mental or social ventures.
old: A perception of the archaic or traditional.

P

penis: Masculinity; a perception of distinctly masculine mental or social qualities; male sexuality. (See **genitalia.**)
physician: (See **doctor.**)
picture: A fixed perception; a memory.
pig: Overindulgent nature or behavior. (See **animal.**)
pimples: A perception of personal imperfection; imperfection of personality.
plants: Perceptions rooted in reality.
police: A perception of moral authority; a implication of blame or guilt; a perception of oppression.
pregnancy: A perception of inner transformation; an inner transformation as a result of a developing social bond. (See **baby** and **birth.**)
president: A personage of social leadership.
profanity: An expression of disrespect.

R

rain: Despair; sadness; a gloomy social perspective.
rape: A profound violation of intimacy and trust. (See **sexual intercourse.**)
rat: Infidelity; unfaithful nature or behavior. (See **animals** and **mouse.**)
restaurant: A inwardly satisfying social experience.
restroom: A public venue where the purging of pent-up thoughts or emotions is appropriate. (See **bathroom, defecation, feces, toilet, urination,** and **urine.**)
road: A mental or social path. (See **ground.**)
robbery: A perception of an unjust or unfair exchange; injustice. (See **bandit.**)
rocks: Impediments. (See **mountain.**)
room: A mental or social experience suggested by the nature of the room.
running: A mental or social effort pursued with urgency to either escape or reach some represented influence or objective. (See **chased.**)

S

school: A learning experience; a environment of structured mental and social experiences.

sea: (See **ocean**.)

sexual intercourse: An exchange of the intimacy and trust that produces social bonds. (See **rape**.)

shark: Opportunistic behavior within a social venture. (See **animals** and **ocean**.)

skinhead: Obtuse; biased; deliberately thoughtless. (See **hair**.)

skunk: A perception of foul behavior; a smelly disposition.

sky: A perception of experiences and influences beyond the usual or mundane; that which is beyond physical experience; a perception of something beyond or ascended.

sleeping: A perception of contentment; obliviousness.

snake: Insidiousness; surreptitious nature or behavior. (See **animals**.)

soldier: A conformist; a perception of social conformity; oppression. (See **military**.)

space: A perception of experience beyond physical reality.

spider: Creepiness; an irrational fear.

spouse: A comforting social influence; a perspective of social comfort and belonging.

store: A mental or social resource.

storm: Rage; social turbulence.

street: (See **road**.)

stuffed animals: Tacit aggression.

sun: An ultimate source of social warmth, clarity, and enlightenment.

T

table: A perception of the interest that is central to some meaningful exchange.

tall: A perception of the respect or prominence of the represented mental or social influence.

tears: A perception of sincere regret.

teeth: Personal beliefs or convictions.

telekinesis: A perception of transcendent mental or social will.

telepathy: A perception of the capacity to understand the thoughts of others.

telephone: A perception of the indirect mental or social means by which one may communicate with another; a perception of indirect communication.

toilet: An appropriate outlet for rancorous mental or emotional purging. (See **bathroom, defecation, feces, restroom, urination,** and **urine**.)

tornado: A turbulence social change. (See **wind**.)
toy: A reference to childlike distraction.
tree: A perception that is firmly rooted in reality.

U

underwater: Overwhelmed; an overwhelming experience.
urination: A mental or emotional purging; purging of frustration or inner turmoil.
urine: Frustration; mental or emotional turmoil.

V

vagina: Femininity; a perception of distinctly feminine mental or social qualities; female sexuality.
vampire: A joyless personage who thrives on the fear and misery of others.
voodoo: An bewitching mental or social influence.

W

wall: A mental or social obstruction or divide.
war: A perception of profound social conflict.
wash: An effort to prepare; a cleansing experience.
water: A meaningful, cleansing, and inwardly satisfying mental or social influence.
wealth: Esteem.
wedding: (See **marriage**.)
werewolf: Inhumane, unsympathetic social behavior.
wind: Social change. (See **tornado**.)
window: A mental or social perspective or outlook.
winter: An inhospitable social climate. (See **cold**.)
wolf: Ruthlessness; avaricious behavior.

Z

zoo: A perspective of the uncivilized, vulgar, and inhumane behaviors kept under social restraint. (See **animals**.)

Notes

Introduction

1. Freud, S., Brill, A. A. *The Interpretation of Dreams.* London: Allen & Unwin, 1915; New York: Macmillan.

GLOSSARY

Afferent. The direction and path sensory information travels into the brain.

Atonia. The state of body musculature characterized by the absence of elasticity.

Atonic sleep. The stage of sleep or restful inactivity characterized by the diversion of energy away from body musculature, causing a loss of muscle tone.

Cerebrum. Cortex.

CNS. Central nervous system.

Conscious. Arousal and awareness in physical reality. The state of wakefulness in the brain characterized by the experience of physical reality through an active and healthy metencephalon.

Consciousness. Relative to dream content, the aspect of awareness that travels between mental and physical experience.

Dreaming. The wakeful activity within the brain aroused by atonic sleep that produces the faux experience of sensory perception and influence.

Dreams. The faux experience of sensory perception and influence suggestive of the psychological influences aroused in the brain by atonic sleep; mental experiences without the distinction of true sensory contact with physical reality.

D-sleep. Dysynchronous sleep. The state of brain activity during atonic sleep that is characterized by low-amplitude, high-frequency EEG waveform patterns and muscle atonia.

EEG. Electroencephalograph.

Efferent. The direction and path CNS directives travel away from the brain.

EMG. Electromyogram.

Endocasts. A mold of the brain made from its cranial casing.

Eukaryote. An organism composed of genetic material surrounded by a membrane forming a nucleus. It is the basis for all animal, plant, and fungal life.

Mental experience. An experience within the environment of cognitive activity aroused by brain function. (See **Mind.**)

Mind. The environment of cognitive activity, within the brain, arising from brain function.

NREM. Non-rapid eye movement.

Perception. The moment of detection, within the brain, of sensory influence.

Phantom-limb syndrome. The persistence of sensory sensation in the rostral stump after a limb has been severed.

Physical experience. An experience with the distinction of sensory contact with physical reality through an active and healthy metencephalon.

Preparation. The surgical procedure by which an animal is prepared for research or study.

Proto-brain. The stage of brain development at the thalamus level in early animals, precursory to current neocortical structure.

Proto-sleep. The stage of sleep development early animals engaged in that involved restful behavior which did not include dreaming. Early animals adapted this behavior, precursory to S-sleep, to conserve energy.

REM. Rapid eye movement.

S-sleep. Synchronous sleep. The state of sleep, associated with NREM sleep, that is characterized by high-amplitude, low-frequency EEG waveform patterns and persistent muscle tone.

Tonic sleep. The stage of sleep or restful inactivity characterized by persistent muscle tone.

Unconscious. Relative to dreaming, the state of brain activity without the distinction of an active or healthy metencephalon. An inactive or unhealthy metencephalon isolates the brain from contact with physicality. Arousal of the brain in isolation from its physical senses creates this surreal state of awareness.

INDEX

978-0-595-37261-4
0-595-37261-9